The Organic Budget Cookbook 2022

Over 100 QuickRecipes and 30-Day Meal Plan

Ricardo A. Adams

Contents

Chapter One

CHICKEN THAT IS SUGARY, STICKY, AND SPICY

Servings: four. - 10 minutes for preparation, 12 minutes for cooking, a total of 22 minutes. FACTS ABOUT DIET AND FITNESS

Total caloric intake (calories plus carbohydrates plus protein plus cholesterol): 232.4

1/4 cup soy sauce 4 skinless, boneless chicken breast halves cut into 1/2 inch strips 2 teaspoons fresh ginger root chopped 1 tablespoon vegetable oil 2 teaspoons minced garlic INGREDIENTS 1 tablespoon brown sugar 2 tablespoons hot sauce 1 tablespoon honey 1 pinch salt and pepper to taste DIRECTIONS

The following ingredients should be combined in a small bowl: brown sugar; honey; soy sauce; ginger; garlic; and hot sauce. 2. Season the chicken strips with a little salt and pepper.

3. In a large skillet, heat the oil over medium heat. About a minute on each side of the chicken strips should be done in the hot oil.

per team. Chicken should be covered in the sauce. To thicken the sauce, cover and cook for 8 to 10 minutes on low heat.

Toasted French bread that is light and airy

The number of servings is 12 Total preparation time is 30 minutes. FACTS ABOUT DIET AND FITNESS

Carbohydrates: 19.4g, Fat: 2.7g, Protein: 4.8g, and Cholesterol: 48mg per serving

INGREDIENTS

2 teaspoons baking powder 1 tablespoon all-purpose flour

cinnamon powder, about a half a teaspoon

8oz. of water

a teaspoon of vanilla flavoring

1 dash of salt

1 tbsp. sugar, white

Three eggs

There are 12 large slices of bread.

DIRECTIONS

In a large bowl, add the flour and mix thoroughly. In a slow, steady stream, add the milk. Eggs and cinnamon are incorporated into the mixture with the salt.

Mix together the sugar and vanilla extract until smooth.

Griddle or fry pans should be heated to medium-high heat.

Soak the bread slices in the mixture for a few minutes, until they are thoroughly moistened. Each side of the bread should be browned. Serve at once.

BIG DADDY BISCUITS are J.P.'s

How many portions are there? 30-minutes of prep time, followed by 15-minutes of cooking time. FACTS ABOUT DIET AND FITNESS

Carbohydrates: 36.4g, Fat: 12.6g, Protein: 5.6g, Cholesterol: 3mg, per serving.

INGREDIENTS

2 quarts of all-purpose wheat flour.

1 tbsp. sugar, white

1-teaspoon powdered sugar

3 tablespoons of shortening

One teaspoon of salt

8oz. of water

DIRECTIONS

Ensure that the oven is set to 425 degrees Fahrenheit (220 degrees C).

Pour all of the ingredients into a large bowl and mix thoroughly. the shortening in half, then

The mixture resembles fine meal. When the dough begins to separate from the bowl, gradually add milk. Knead 15 to 20 times on a floured surface before forming into a ball. Dough should be rolled or patted out to a thickness of 1 inch. You can use a large cutter or juice glass that has been dusted in flour to make biscuits. To finish, keep going until all of the dough is used up. On an ungreased baking sheet, brush off any excess flour, then place the biscuits in the oven to bake.

Bake for 13 to 15 minutes, or until the edges begin to brown, in a preheated oven.

SUCCESSFUL, TASTY TURKEY BURGER SALAD

The number of servings is 12 - 15m Prep - 15m Cooking - Total: 30m. Nutrition Facts: 183 calories, 2.3 grams of carbohydrates, 9.5 grams of fat, 20.9 grams of protein, and 90 milligrams of cholesterol.

INGREDIENTS: 3 pounds of ground turkey; 1/4 cup chopped fresh parsley; 1/4 cup seasoned bread crumbs; 1 peeled and minced garlic clove; 1/4 cup finely diced onion; 1 teaspoon salt; 2 lightly beaten egg whites; 1/4 teaspoon ground black pepper.

Pour all of the ingredients for the meatloaf into a large bowl and mix thoroughly.

pepper. Make 12 patties out of the mixture.

Over medium heat, cook the patties until they reach an internal temperature of 180 degrees F by turning them once (85 degrees C).

Asparagus baked in a BALSAMIC BUTTER SAUCE.

Servings: four. - Prep: 10m - Cooks: 12m - Total: 25m - Additional: 3m - FACTS ABOUT DIET AND FITNESS Carbohydrates: 4.9g; Fat: 5.9g; Protein: 2.8g; Cholesterol: 15mg. 2 tablespoons butter f cooking spray f 1 tablespoon soy sauce f salt and pepper to taste f 1 teaspoon balsamic vinegar

DIRECTIONS

The oven should be preheated to 400 degrees Fahrenheit (200 degrees C).

A baking sheet should be used to arrange the asparagus in an attractive fashion. Add salt and pepper to taste and spray with cooking spray. The asparagus will be ready after 12 minutes in a preheated oven.

Cook the butter in a medium-sized pot until it is completely melted. Remove from the heat and add balsamic vinegar and soy sauce to the pan.

vinegar. Serve with the asparagus that has been baked.

AN EASY CASSEROLE FROM MEXICO

How many portions are there? - Preparation: 20m - Cooking: 30m - Total: 50m FACTS ABOUT DIET AND FITNESS

632 calories, 32.8 grams of carbohydrates, 43.7 grams of fat, 31.7 grams of protein, and 119 milligrams of cholesterol.

The ingredients include 1 pound of lean ground beef, 2 cups of salsa, 1/2 cup of chopped green onion, 1 pound of chili beans, and 3 cups of crushed tortilla chips, as well as 2 cups of Cheddar cheese and 2 cup of sour cream, per serving. DIRECTIONS

Make sure the oven is preheated to 350 degrees Fahrenheit (175 degrees C).

Ground beef should no longer be pink when cooked in a large skillet over medium-high heat. Simmer the salsa for a few minutes before serving.

When the liquid has been absorbed, turn down the heat and simmer for another 20 minutes. Make sure they're all heated through. Cooking spray can be used to coat a 9x13 baking dish. Spread a layer of crushed tortilla chips on the bottom of the dish, followed by a layer of beef mixture. To serve, top beef with sour cream and a medley of olives, green onion, and tomato. Add a sprinkling of shredded Cheddar cheese to the top.

When it's hot and bubbly, take it out of the oven and serve.

Pork chops seasoned with Italian herbs and spices.

Servings: four. - Preparation time: 25 minutes; cooking time: 35 minutes; total cooking time: one hour. The following are the nutrition facts for one serving: 440 calories, 33.4% carbohydrates, 20% fat, 30% protein, and 186 mg cholesterol.

RECIPE INGREDIENTS: 3 light-beaten eggs; 3 tablespoons milk, 2 tablespoons olive oil, 2 tablespoons dried parsley, and a pinch of salt and pepper One-half cup Bread crumbs flavored with Italian seasoning f Garlic cloves: 4 peeled and chopped cloves A half cup of finely grated Parmesan cheese Pork chops in fours

DIRECTIONS

325 degrees Fahrenheit is the ideal temperature for baking (160 degrees C).

Beat the eggs and milk together in a small bowl. In a separate bowl, combine the bread crumbs and seasonings.

Parsley and Parmesan cheese.

Using an oven-safe skillet, heat the olive oil to medium-high in a large saucepan. Add the garlic and cook for a few minutes until it's a little browned. Remove the garlic and save it for later use.

Coat each pork chop evenly by dipping it in the egg mixture and then in the bread crumb mixture.

Brown each side of the pork chops for about five minutes.

To achieve an internal temperature of 145 degrees Fahrenheit, cook the pork chops in a skillet for 25 minutes (63 degrees C).

Astonishing CHICKEN!

How many portions are there? Total time: 9 hours and 25 minutes, including prep time and cooking time. NUTRITIONAL DATA Calories 337.1, Carbohydrates 22.4g, Protein 24.8g, Cholesterol 67.1 mg.

INGREDIENTS: 1/4 cup cider vinegar, 1/2 cup brown sugar, 3 tablespoons prepared coarse-ground mustard, 1 1/2 teaspoons salt, 3 minced garlic cloves, 1 teaspoon freshly ground black pepper, 1 lime juiced, 6 tablespoons olive oil, 1/2 lemon juice, 6 skinless, boneless chicken breast halves.

DIRECTIONS

Pour the cider vinegar, mustard, garlic, lime juice, lemon juice, brown sugar, salt, and pepper into a large glass bowl.

as well as salt and pepper. Add the olive oil and mix. Add the chicken to the mix. Cover and marinate for 8 hours or overnight.

Outdoor grills should be preheated to a high temperature before use.

Grill grates should be brushed with a light coating of oil. Cook the chicken for 6 to 8 minutes on each side on the preheated grill, or until the juices run clear when pierced with a fork. Toss out the marinade.

Lime and Garlic Tilapia

Servings: four. - 10 minutes for preparation, 30 minutes for cooking, a total of 40 minutes. FACTS ABOUT DIET AND FITNESS

Fat: 4.4g; Protein: 23.1g; Cholesterol: 49mg; 142 calories.

INGREDIENTS: 4 tilapia fillets; 1 minced clove of garlic; 3 tablespoons fresh lemon juice; 1 teaspoon dried parsley flakes; 1 tablespoon butter; freshly ground pepper;

DIRECTIONS

Start by preheating the oven to 375°F (190 degrees C). A baking pan should be sprayed with non-stick cooking spray. In order to remove any excess moisture, pat the fillets dry with paper towels.

The fillets should be placed in a baking dish. Sprinkle butter on top of lemon juice before serving. Add some minced garlic to the mix.

pepper and parsley.

Cook the fish in a preheated oven until it is white and flaky, about 30 minutes.

CHICKEN NUGGETS BAKED IN A PAN

How many portions are there? - Prep: 20 minutes; Cooks: 20 minutes; Total: 40 minutes. Nutrition Facts: Calories: 308, Carbohydrates: 14.6g, Protein: 19.3g, Cholesterol: 81mg 1 teaspoon dried thyme 1 cup seasoned Italian breadcrumbs 1 tablespoon dried basil 1/2 cup Parmesan cheese melted in butter 1 teaspoon salt Ingredients: 3 skinless, boneless chicken breasts DIRECTIONS

The oven should be preheated to 400 degrees Fahrenheit (200 degrees C).

1 1/2-inch cubes of chicken breasts, cut in half crosswise. The bread crumbs and butter should be combined in a medium bowl.

cheese, thyme, salt, and basil Make sure everything is well combined. Dip a piece of bread in a bowl of melted butter before serving. Dip the chicken pieces in the melted butter, then in the breadcrumb mixture, to coat them completely.

Bake the well-coated chicken for 20 minutes on a cookie sheet lightly greased with cooking spray.

SAUTEED APPLES

Servings: 8 - Prep: 5m - Cooks: 15m - Total: 20m FACTS ABOUT DIET AND FITNESS

Calories: 143, Carbohydrates: 24.3g, Fat: 5.9g, Protein: 0.4g, Cholesterol: 15mg

INGREDIENTS\sf 1/4 cup butter\sf 1/2 cup cold water\sf 4 large tart apples - peeled, cored and sliced 1/4 inch thick\sf 1/2cup brown sugar\sf 2 teaspoons cornstarch\sf 1/2teaspoon ground cinnamon

DIRECTIONS

In a large skillet or saucepan, melt butter over medium heat; add apples. Cook, stirring constantly, until

apples are almost tender, about 6 to 7 minutes.

Dissolve cornstarch in water; add to skillet. Stir in brown sugar and cinnamon. Boil for 2 minutes, stirring occasionally. Remove from heat and serve warm.

A GOOD EASY GARLIC CHICKEN

Servings: four. - Prep: 10m - Cooks: 10m - Total: 20m NUTRITION FACTS\sCalories: 213.8, Carbohydrates: 1.7g, Protein: 27.6g, Cholesterol: 91.3mg

INGREDIENTS\sf 3 tablespoons butter\sf 1 teaspoon seasoning salt\sf 4 skinless, boneless chicken breast halves\sf 1 teaspoon onion powder f 2 teaspoons garlic powder

DIRECTIONS

1. Melt butter in a large skillet over medium high heat. Add chicken and sprinkle with garlic powder,

seasoning salt and onion powder. Saute about 10 to 15 minutes on each side, or until chicken is cooked through and juices run clear.

EASY TUNA CASSEROLE

Servings: 8 - Prep: 15m - Cooks: 30m - Total: 45m FACTS ABOUT DIET AND FITNESS

Calories: 462, Carbohydrates: 37.1g, Fat: 28.5g, Protein: 11.5g, Cholesterol: 23mg

INGREDIENTS\sf 3 cups cooked macaroni\sf 1 cup shredded Cheddar cheese f 1 (5 ounce) can tuna, drained f 1 1/2 cups French fried onions\sf 1 (10.75 ounce) can condensed cream of chicken soup

DIRECTIONS

Make sure the oven is preheated to 350 degrees Fahrenheit (175 degrees C).

In a 9x13-inch baking dish, combine the macaroni, tuna, and soup. Mix well, and then top with cheese. 3. Bake at 350 degrees F (175 degrees C) for about 25 minutes, or until bubbly. Sprinkle with fried onions,

and bake for another 5 minutes. Serve at once.

FRENCH TOAST CASSEROLE

How many portions are there? - Prep: 30m - Cooks: 50m - Total: 1h20m NUTRITION FACTS\sCalories: 207, Carbohydrates: 26.6g, Fat: 7.2g, Protein: 8.5g, Cholesterol: 129mg

INGREDIENTS\sf 5 cups bread cubes f 1/4 teaspoon salt f 4 eggs\sf 1 teaspoon vanilla extract\sf 1 1/2 cups milk\sf 1 tablespoon margarine, softened\sf 1/4 cup white sugar, divided f 1 teaspoon ground cinnamon DIRECTIONS

1. Preheat oven to 350 degrees F (175 degrees C) (175 degrees C). Lightly butter an 8x8 inch baking pan. 2. Line bottom of pan with bread cubes. In a large bowl, beat together eggs, milk, 2 tablespoons sugar, salt

and vanilla. pour egg mixture over bread. Dot with margarine; let stand for 10 minutes. 3.\sCombine remaining 2 tablespoons sugar with 1 teaspoon cinnamon and sprinkle over the top.

Bake in\spreheated oven about 45 to 50 minutes, until top is golden.

SOUR CREAM PORK CHOPS

How many portions are there? - Prep: 15m - Cooks: 8h30m - Total: 8h45m FACTS ABOUT DIET AND FITNESS

Calories: 257, Carbohydrates: 14.3g, Fat: 14.4g, Protein: 16.8g, Cholesterol: 54mg

INGREDIENTS f 6 pork chops f 2 cubes chicken bouillon f salt and pepper to taste f 2 cups boiling water f garlic powder to taste f 2 tablespoons all-purpose flour f 1/2 cup all-purpose flour f 1 (8 ounce) container sour cream f 1 large onion, sliced 1/4 inch thick DIRECTIONS Season pork chops with salt, pepper, and garlic powder, and then dredge in 1/2 cup flour. In a skillet

over medium heat, lightly brown chops in a small amount of oil.

Place chops in slow cooker, and top with onion slices. Dissolve bouillon cubes in boiling water and pour over chops. Cover, and cook on Low 7 to 8 hours.

Preheat oven to 200 degrees F (95 degrees C).

After the chops have cooked, transfer chops to the oven to keep warm. Be careful, the chops are so tender they will fall apart. In a small bowl, blend 2 tablespoons flour with the sour cream; mix into meat juices. Turn slow cooker to High for 15 to 30 minutes, or until sauce is slightly thickened. Serve sauce over pork chops.

SLOW COOKER LEMON GARLIC CHICKEN

How many portions are there? - Prep: 15m - Cooks: 3h15m - Total: 3h30m NUTRITION FACTS Calories: 192.3, Carbohydrates: 1.3g , Protein: 29.6g, Cholesterol: 88.2mg

INGREDIENTS f 1 teaspoon dried oregano f 1/4 cup water f 1/2 teaspoon salt f 3 tablespoons fresh lemon juice f 1/4 teaspoon ground black pepper f 2 cloves garlic, minced f 2 pounds skinless, boneless chicken breast halves f 1 teaspoon chicken bouillon granules f 2 tablespoons butter f 1 teaspoon chopped fresh parsley

DIRECTIONS

In a bowl, mix the oregano, salt, and pepper. Rub the mixture into chicken. Melt the butter in a skillet

over medium heat. Brown chicken in butter for 3 to 5 minutes on each side. Place chicken in a slow cooker.

In the same skillet, mix the water, lemon juice, garlic, and bouillon. Bring the mixture to boil. Pour over the chicken in the slow cooker.

Cover, and cook on High for 3 hours, or Low for 6 hours. Add the parsley to the slow cooker 15 to 30 minutes before the end of the cook time.

GREEK CHICKEN PASTA

How many portions are there? - 15m Prep - 15m Cooking - Total: 30m. FACTS ABOUT DIET AND FITNESS

Calories: 487.7, Carbohydrates: 70g , Protein: 32.6g, Cholesterol: 55mg

INGREDIENTS f 1 (16 ounce) package linguine pasta f 1/2 cup crumbled feta cheese f 1/2 cup chopped red onion f 3 tablespoons chopped fresh parsley f 1 tablespoon olive oil f 2 tablespoons lemon juice f 2 cloves garlic, crushed f 2 teaspoons dried oregano f 1 pound skinless, boneless chicken breast meat - cut into bite-size pieces f salt and pepper to taste f 1 (14 ounce) can marinated artichoke hearts, drained and chopped f 2 lemons, wedged, for garnish f 1 large tomato, chopped DIRECTIONS Bring a large pot of lightly salted water to a boil. Cook pasta in boiling water until tender yet firm to the

bit, 8 to 10 minutes; drain.

Heat olive oil in a large skillet over medium-high heat. Add onion and garlic; saute until fragrant, about 2 minutes. Stir in the chicken and cook, stirring occasionally, until chicken is no longer pink in the center and the juices run clear, about 5 to 6 minutes.

Reduce heat to medium-low; add artichoke hearts, tomato, feta cheese, parsley, lemon juice, oregano, and cooked pasta. Cook and stir until heated through, about 2 to 3 minutes.

Remove from heat, season with salt and pepper, and garnish with lemon wedges.

VEGETARIAN CHICKPEA SANDWICH FILLING

Servings: 3 - Prep: 20m - Cooks: 0m - Total: 20m FACTS ABOUT DIET AND FITNESS

Calories: 259, Carbohydrates: 43.5g, Fat: 5.8g, Protein: 9.3g, Cholesterol: 2mg

INGREDIENTS f 1 (19 ounce) can garbanzo beans, drained and rinsed f 1 tablespoon lemon juice f 1 stalk celery, chopped f 1 teaspoon dried dill weed f 1/2 onion, chopped f salt and pepper to taste f 1 tablespoon mayonnaise DIRECTIONS 1. Drain and rinse chickpeas. Pour chickpeas into a medium size mixing bowl and mash with a fork. Mix in

celery, onion, mayonnaise (to taste), lemon juice, dill, salt and pepper to taste. Watch Now.

SPICY BEAN SALSA

The number of servings is 12 - Prep: 10m - Cooks: 8h - Total: 8h10m - Additional: 8h NUTRITION FACTS Calories: 155, Carbohydrates: 20.4g, Fat: 6.4g, Protein: 5g, Cholesterol: 0mg

INGREDIENTS f 1 (15 ounce) can black-eyed peas f 1 (4 ounce) can diced jalapeno peppers f 1 (15 ounce) can black beans, rinsed and drained f 1 (14.5 ounce) can diced tomatoes, drained f 1 (15 ounce) can whole kernel corn, drained f 1 cup Italian-style salad dressing f 1/2 cup chopped onion f 1/2 teaspoon garlic salt f 1/2 cup chopped green bell pepper

DIRECTIONS 1. In a medium bowl, combine black-eyed peas, black beans, corn, onion, green bell pepper, jalapeno

peppers and tomatoes. Season with Italian-style salad dressing and garlic salt; mix well. Cover, and refrigerate overnight to blend flavors.

KEY WEST CHICKEN

Servings: four. - Prep: 15m - Cooks: 15m - Total: 1h - Additional: 30m FACTS ABOUT DIET AND FITNESS

Calories: 184.1, Carbohydrates: 5.6g, Protein: 25.3g, Cholesterol: 67.2mg

INGREDIENTS

◆ 3 tablespoons soy sauce

◆ 1 teaspoon lime juice

◆ 1 tablespoon honey ◆ 1 teaspoon chopped garlic

◆ 1 tablespoon vegetable oil

◆ 4 skinless, boneless chicken breast halves

DIRECTIONS

In a shallow container, blend soy sauce, honey, vegetable oil, lime juice, and garlic. Place chicken breast halves into the mixture, and turn to coat. Cover, and marinate in the refrigerator at least 30 minutes.

Outdoor grills should be preheated to a high temperature before use.

Grill grates should be brushed with a light coating of oil. Discard marinade, and grill chicken 6 to 8 minutes on each side, until juices run clear.

QUICK CHICKEN PICCATA

Servings: four. - Prep: 10m - Cooks: 15m - Total: 25m
NUTRITION FACTS Calories: 320.6, Carbohydrates: 8.4g, Protein: 24.7g, Cholesterol: 87.5mg INGREDIENTS f 4 eaches skinless, boneless chicken breast halves f 1/2 cup white wine f 1 pinch cayenne pepper, or to taste f 1/4 cup fresh lemon juice f 1 pinch salt and ground black pepper to taste f 1/4 cup water f 1/4 cup all-purpose flour for dredging f 3 tablespoons cold unsalted butter, cut in 1/4-inch slices f 2 tablespoons olive oil f 2 tablespoons fresh Italian parsley, chopped f 1 tablespoon capers, drained DIRECTIONS

1. Place chicken breasts between 2 layers of plastic wrap and pound to about 1/2-inch thick. 2. Season both sides of chicken breasts with cayenne, salt, and black pepper; dredge lightly in flour and

shake off any excess.

3. Heat olive oil in a skillet over medium-high heat. Place chicken in the pan, reduce heat to medium, and cook until browned and cooked through, about 5 minutes per side; remove to a plate. 4. Cook capers in reserved oil, smashing them lightly to release brine, until warmed though, about 30 seconds.

Pour white wine into skillet. Scrape any browned bits from the bottom of the pan with a wooden spoon.

Cook until reduced by half, about 2 minutes.

Stir lemon juice, water, and butter into the reduced wine mixture; cook and stir continuously to form a thick sauce, about 2 minutes. Reduce heat to low and stir parsley through the sauce. 7. Return chicken breasts to the pan cook until heated through, 1 to 2 minutes. Serve with sauce spooned over the top.

muffins with bananas, oatmeal, and maple syrup

The number of servings: 12. - Preparation: 15m - Cooking: 20m - Total: 35m - A FEW FACTS ABOUT DIET

The calorie count is 200. Carbohydrates: 30.1g, Fat: 7.5g, Protein: 3.7g, Cholesterol: 17mg.

All-purpose flour, unbleached, 1 egg, and salt Oatmeal, milk, white sugar, and vegetable oil are all mixed together in a single cup. 2-teaspoon flour, 1/2-teaspoon vanilla, 1-teaspoon baking soda, 1-cup bananas, 1/2-teaspoon salt: this is what you'll need. DIRECTIONS

Add flour, oats, sugar, baking powder, soda, and salt to a bowl.

Briskly whisk the egg whites in a large bowl. Add the milk, oil, and vanilla. Add the mashed banana and thoroughly mix it into the batter. Just before serving, stir in the flour mixture. Using paper baking cups, divide the batter among the 12 muffin tins.

To cook, preheat the oven to 400°F (205°C).

Incredible chicken

4 - 10 minutes for preparation - 30 minutes for cooking - 40 minutes total A FEW FACTS ABOUT DIET

547.8 kcal, 40.9 g carbs, 32.8 g protein, and 77.6 mg cholesterol are the caloric totals.

This recipe calls for four chicken breast halves that are skinless and boneless, as well as one teaspoon each of salt and pepper to taste, as well as two cups of Italian breadcrumbs.

DIRECTIONS

Pre-heat your oven to 425°F. Clean and butter a small baking dish. 2. Salt and pepper chicken breasts. Mayonnaise-coated chicken is rolled in bread crumbs until it's evenly coated on all sides.

coated. Add coated breasts to the pan and bake as directed.

To make sure the chicken is cooked through but still moist, bake it uncovered for 30 minutes at 375°F.

CURRY OF RED LENTILS

The number of servings: 12. - 10 minutes for preparation - 30 minutes for cooking - 40 minutes total A FEW FACTS ABOUT DIET

192 calories, 32.5 grams of carbohydrates, 2.6 grams of fat, 12.1 grams of protein, and 0mg of cholesterol.

INGREDIENTS

2 mugs of red lentil soup

Chilli powder in the amount of 1 teaspoon

Diced onion, about 1 large one

Salt, white sugar, and one tablespoon of vegetable oil are the only ingredients you'll need.

2 tblsp. curry powder

This recipe calls for 1 teaspoon of minced garlic

One-fourth cup ground coriander

Ginger minced with a knife

1 tsp. turmeric powder

one 14.25-ounce can of pureed tomato

1 tbsp. cumin seed powder.

DIRECTIONS

In a bowl, combine the lentils, water, and salt; stir to combine. Pour water over the lentils in a pot and bring to a boil.

Simmer on medium-low heat for 15 to 20 minutes, adding water as needed to keep the pot covered, until the vegetables are tender. Drain.

Over medium heat, cook and stir onions in a large skillet until they are caramelized, about 20 minutes; drain and set aside.

Then, in a large bowl, combine the onion mixture with the curry paste and all of the other ingredients except the chili powder (including the salt, sugar, garlic, and ginger). Turn the heat up to high and cook for 1 to 2 minutes, stirring constantly, until the mixture is fragrant.

Immediately after removing from the heat, stir in the tomato puree.

Chapter Two

SOUR CREAM PORK CHOPS

How many portions are there? - Prep: 15m - Cooks: 8h30m - Total: 8h45m FACTS ABOUT DIET AND FITNESS

Calories: 257, Carbohydrates: 14.3g, Fat: 14.4g, Protein: 16.8g, Cholesterol: 54mg

INGREDIENTS f 6 pork chops f 2 cubes chicken bouillon f salt and pepper to taste f 2 cups boiling water f garlic powder to taste f 2 tablespoons all-purpose flour f 1/2 cup all-purpose flour f 1 (8 ounce) container sour cream f 1 large onion, sliced 1/4 inch thick DIRECTIONS Season pork chops with salt, pepper, and garlic powder, and then dredge in 1/2 cup flour. In a skillet

over medium heat, lightly brown chops in a small amount of oil.

Place chops in slow cooker, and top with onion slices. Dissolve bouillon cubes in boiling water and pour over chops. Cover, and cook on Low 7 to 8 hours.

Preheat oven to 200 degrees F (95 degrees C).

After the chops have cooked, transfer chops to the oven to keep warm. Be careful, the chops are so tender they will fall apart. In a small bowl, blend 2 tablespoons flour with the sour cream; mix into meat juices. Turn slow cooker to High for 15 to 30 minutes, or until sauce is slightly thickened. Serve sauce over pork chops.

SLOW COOKER LEMON GARLIC CHICKEN

How many portions are there? - Prep: 15m - Cooks: 3h15m - Total: 3h30m NUTRITION FACTS Calories: 192.3, Carbohydrates: 1.3g , Protein: 29.6g, Cholesterol: 88.2mg

INGREDIENTS f 1 teaspoon dried oregano f 1/4 cup water f 1/2 teaspoon salt f 3 tablespoons fresh lemon juice f 1/4 teaspoon ground black pepper f 2 cloves garlic, minced f 2 pounds skinless, boneless chicken breast halves f 1 teaspoon chicken bouillon granules f 2 tablespoons butter f 1 teaspoon chopped fresh parsley

DIRECTIONS

In a bowl, mix the oregano, salt, and pepper. Rub the mixture into chicken. Melt the butter in a skillet over medium heat. Brown chicken in butter for 3 to 5 minutes on each side. Place chicken in a slow cooker.

In the same skillet, mix the water, lemon juice, garlic, and bouillon. Bring the mixture to boil. Pour over the chicken in the slow cooker.

Cover, and cook on High for 3 hours, or Low for 6 hours. Add the parsley to the slow cooker 15 to 30 minutes before the end of the cook time.

GREEK CHICKEN PASTA

How many portions are there? - 15m Prep - 15m Cooking - Total: 30m. FACTS ABOUT DIET AND FITNESS

Calories: 487.7, Carbohydrates: 70g , Protein: 32.6g, Cholesterol: 55mg

INGREDIENTS f 1 (16 ounce) package linguine pasta f 1/2 cup crumbled feta cheese f 1/2 cup chopped red onion f 3 tablespoons chopped fresh parsley f 1 tablespoon olive oil f 2 tablespoons lemon juice f 2 cloves garlic, crushed f 2 teaspoons dried oregano f 1 pound skinless, boneless chicken breast meat - cut into bite-size pieces f salt and pepper to taste f 1 (14 ounce) can marinated artichoke hearts, drained and chopped f 2 lemons, wedged, for garnish f 1 large tomato, chopped DIRECTIONS Bring a large pot of lightly salted water to a boil. Cook pasta in boiling water until tender yet firm to the bit, 8 to 10 minutes; drain.

Heat olive oil in a large skillet over medium-high heat. Add onion and garlic; saute until fragrant, about 2 minutes. Stir in the chicken and cook, stirring occasionally, until chicken is no longer pink in the center and the juices run clear, about 5 to 6 minutes.

Reduce heat to medium-low; add artichoke hearts, tomato, feta cheese, parsley, lemon juice, oregano, and cooked pasta. Cook and stir until heated through, about 2 to 3 minutes. Remove from heat, season with salt and pepper, and garnish with lemon wedges.

VEGETARIAN CHICKPEA SANDWICH FILLING

Servings: 3 - Prep: 20m - Cooks: 0m - Total: 20m FACTS ABOUT DIET AND FITNESS

Calories: 259, Carbohydrates: 43.5g, Fat: 5.8g, Protein: 9.3g, Cholesterol: 2mg

INGREDIENTS f 1 (19 ounce) can garbanzo beans, drained and rinsed f 1 tablespoon lemon juice f 1 stalk celery, chopped f 1 teaspoon dried dill weed f 1/2 onion, chopped f salt and pepper to taste f 1 tablespoon mayonnaise DIRECTIONS 1. Drain and rinse chickpeas. Pour chickpeas into a medium size mixing bowl and mash with a fork. Mix in celery, onion, mayonnaise (to taste), lemon juice, dill, salt and pepper to taste. Watch Now.

SPICY BEAN SALSA

The number of servings is 12 - Prep: 10m - Cooks: 8h - Total: 8h10m - Additional: 8h NUTRITION FACTS Calories: 155, Carbohydrates: 20.4g, Fat: 6.4g, Protein: 5g, Cholesterol: 0mg

INGREDIENTS f 1 (15 ounce) can black-eyed peas f 1 (4 ounce) can diced jalapeno peppers f 1 (15 ounce) can black beans, rinsed and drained f 1 (14.5 ounce) can diced tomatoes, drained f 1 (15 ounce) can whole kernel corn, drained f 1 cup Italian-style salad dressing f 1/2 cup chopped onion f 1/2 teaspoon garlic salt f 1/2 cup chopped green bell pepper

DIRECTIONS 1. In a medium bowl, combine black-eyed peas, black beans, corn, onion, green bell pepper, jalapeno

peppers and tomatoes. Season with Italian-style salad dressing and garlic salt; mix well. Cover, and refrigerate overnight to blend flavors.

KEY WEST CHICKEN

Servings: four. - Prep: 15m - Cooks: 15m - Total: 1h - Additional: 30m FACTS ABOUT DIET AND FITNESS

Calories: 184.1, Carbohydrates: 5.6g, Protein: 25.3g, Cholesterol: 67.2mg

INGREDIENTS

- 3 tablespoons soy sauce

- 1 teaspoon lime juice

- 1 tablespoon honey ◆ 1 teaspoon chopped garlic

- 1 tablespoon vegetable oil

- 4 skinless, boneless chicken breast halves

DIRECTIONS

In a shallow container, blend soy sauce, honey, vegetable oil, lime juice, and garlic. Place chicken breast

halves into the mixture, and turn to coat. Cover, and marinate in the refrigerator at least 30 minutes.

Outdoor grills should be preheated to a high temperature before use.

Grill grates should be brushed with a light coating of oil. Discard marinade, and grill chicken 6 to 8 minutes on each side, until juices run clear.

QUICK CHICKEN PICCATA

Servings: four. - Prep: 10m - Cooks: 15m - Total: 25m
NUTRITION FACTS Calories: 320.6, Carbohydrates: 8.4g, Protein: 24.7g, Cholesterol: 87.5mg INGREDIENTS f 4 eaches skinless, boneless chicken breast halves f 1/2 cup white wine f 1 pinch cayenne pepper, or to taste f 1/4 cup fresh lemon juice f 1 pinch salt and ground black pepper to taste f 1/4 cup water

f 1/4 cup all-purpose flour for dredging f 3 tablespoons cold unsalted butter, cut in 1/4-inch slices f 2 tablespoons olive oil f 2 tablespoons fresh Italian parsley, chopped f 1 tablespoon capers, drained DIRECTIONS

1. Place chicken breasts between 2 layers of plastic wrap and pound to about 1/2-inch thick. 2. Season both sides of chicken breasts with cayenne, salt, and black pepper; dredge lightly in flour and

shake off any excess.

3. Heat olive oil in a skillet over medium-high heat. Place chicken in the pan, reduce heat to medium, and cook until browned and cooked through, about 5 minutes per side; remove to a plate. 4. Cook capers in reserved oil, smashing them lightly to release brine, until warmed though, about 30 seconds.

Pour white wine into skillet. Scrape any browned bits from the bottom of the pan with a wooden spoon.

Cook until reduced by half, about 2 minutes.

Stir lemon juice, water, and butter into the reduced wine mixture; cook and stir continuously to form a thick sauce, about 2 minutes. Reduce heat to low and stir parsley through the sauce. 7. Return chicken breasts to the pan cook until heated through, 1 to 2 minutes. Serve with sauce spooned over the top.

muffins with bananas, oatmeal, and maple syrup

The number of servings: 12. - Preparation: 15m - Cooking: 20m - Total: 35m - A FEW FACTS ABOUT DIET

The calorie count is 200. Carbohydrates: 30.1g, Fat: 7.5g, Protein: 3.7g, Cholesterol: 17mg.

All-purpose flour, unbleached, 1 egg, and salt Oatmeal, milk, white sugar, and vegetable oil are all mixed together in a single cup. 2-teaspoon flour, 1/2-teaspoon vanilla, 1-teaspoon baking soda, 1-cup bananas, 1/2-teaspoon salt: this is what you'll need. DIRECTIONS

Add flour, oats, sugar, baking powder, soda, and salt to a bowl.

Briskly whisk the egg whites in a large bowl. Add the milk, oil, and vanilla. Add the mashed banana and thoroughly mix it into the batter. Just before serving, stir in the flour mixture. Using paper baking cups, divide the batter among the 12 muffin tins.

To cook, preheat the oven to 400°F (205°C).

Incredible chicken

4 - 10 minutes for preparation - 30 minutes for cooking - 40 minutes total A FEW FACTS ABOUT DIET

547.8 kcal, 40.9 g carbs, 32.8 g protein, and 77.6 mg cholesterol are the caloric totals.

This recipe calls for four chicken breast halves that are skinless and boneless, as well as one teaspoon each of salt and pepper to taste, as well as two cups of Italian breadcrumbs.

DIRECTIONS

Pre-heat your oven to 425°F. Clean and butter a small baking dish. 2. Salt and pepper chicken breasts. Mayonnaise-coated chicken is rolled in bread crumbs until it's evenly coated on all sides.

coated. Add coated breasts to the pan and bake as directed.

To make sure the chicken is cooked through but still moist, bake it uncovered for 30 minutes at 375°F.

CURRY OF RED LENTILS

The number of servings: 12. - 10 minutes for preparation - 30 minutes for cooking - 40 minutes total A FEW FACTS ABOUT DIET

192 calories, 32.5 grams of carbohydrates, 2.6 grams of fat, 12.1 grams of protein, and 0mg of cholesterol.

INGREDIENTS

2 mugs of red lentil soup

Chilli powder in the amount of 1 teaspoon

Diced onion, about 1 large one

Salt, white sugar, and one tablespoon of vegetable oil are the only ingredients you'll need.

2 tblsp. curry powder

This recipe calls for 1 teaspoon of minced garlic

One-fourth cup ground coriander

Ginger minced with a knife

1 tsp. turmeric powder

one 14.25-ounce can of pureed tomato

1 tbsp. cumin seed powder.

DIRECTIONS

In a bowl, combine the lentils, water, and salt; stir to combine. Pour water over the lentils in a pot and bring to a boil.

Simmer on medium-low heat for 15 to 20 minutes, adding water as needed to keep the pot covered, until the vegetables are tender. Drain.

Over medium heat, cook and stir onions in a large skillet until they are caramelized, about 20 minutes; drain and set aside.

Then, in a large bowl, combine the onion mixture with the curry paste and all of the other ingredients except the chili powder (including the salt, sugar, garlic, and ginger). Turn the heat up to high and cook for 1 to 2 minutes, stirring constantly, until the mixture is fragrant.

Immediately after removing from the heat, stir in the tomato puree.

Chapter Three

ROLLER OF UNSTUFFIED CABBAGE

Servings: Six - Prep: 20m - Cooks: 35m - Total: 55m - Nutrition Facts: 398 calories, 16.3 grams of carbohydrates, 23.8 grams of fat, 28.5 grams of protein, 93 milligrams of cholesterol.

Ingredients include 2 pounds of ground beef, 1/2 cup of water, a large onion, chopped, 2 cloves of garlic, minced, a small head of cabbage, chopped, 2 teaspoons of salt, and 2 (14.5 ounce) cans of diced tomatoes. Over medium-high heat, bring a Dutch oven or large skillet to a boil. Beef and onion are cooked and stirred in a hot Dutch oven.

Remove from the oven and allow to cool for 5 to 7 minutes before draining and discarding the grease. Add cabbage, tomatoes, tomato sauce, water, garlic, salt, and pepper and bring to a boil. Simmer the cabbage for about 30 minutes, covered, on a low heat.

Soup made with beef, barley, and vegetables

At least ten. Preparation: 20 minutes - Cooking: 5h30m - Total: 5h50m A FEW FACTS ABOUT DIET

Calories: 321, Carbohydrates: 22.4g, Fat: 17.3g, Protein: 20g, Cholesterol: 62mg

INGREDIENTS\sf 1 (3 pound) beef chuck roast\sf 4 cups water\sf 1/2 cup barley\sf 4 cubes beef bouillon cube\sf 1 bay leaf\sf 1 tablespoon white sugar\sf 2 tablespoons oil\sf 1/4 teaspoon ground black pepper\sf 3 carrots, chopped\sf 1 (28 ounce) can chopped stewed tomatoes\sf 3 stalks celery, chopped\sf salt to taste\sf 1 onion, chopped\sf ground black pepper to taste\sf 1 (16 ounce) package frozen mixed vegetables

DIRECTIONS

chuck roast should be cooked for at least four to five hours on high in a slow cooker, but this can vary depending on the type of slow cooker.

slow cookers that aren't the same During the final hour of cooking, add barley and bay leaves. Remove the meat from the bones and chop it into small pieces. The bay leaf should be thrown away. Set aside beef, broth, and barley.

Heat oil in a large stock pot over medium-high heat. Fryed mixed vegetables and carrots should be sauteed until they are fork tender. Salt, sugar and 1/4 teaspoon pepper are added to the beef/barley mixture along with the bouillon cubes and water. Simmer for 10 to 20 minutes after bringing to a boil. Add more salt and pepper to your liking, if desired.

Asian Beef with Snow Peas

4 - Prep: 5m - Cooks: 10m - Total: 15m - A FEW FACTS ABOUT DIET

203 calories, 9.7 grams of carbs, 10 grams of fat, and 16 grams of protein. Cholesterol: 39mg

INGREDIENTS

soy sauce, 3 tbsp.

Fresh ginger root, minced, 1 tablespoon

Wine made from rice, 2 tablespoons

1-teaspoon of finely minced garlic

Sugar in the form of granulated brown sugar

Beef round steak, thinly sliced

1/3 cup cornstarch (or similar thickener)

Peas, fresh or frozen, 8 oz.

1 tbsp. oil from vegetable sources

DIRECTIONS

Soy sauce, rice wine, brown sugar, and cornstarch should be combined in a small bowl. Set aside for later use. Pour the oil into a wok or skillet and bring it to a boil over medium heat. 30-second stir-fries of ginger and garlic Then, add the

After 2 minutes, remove the steaks from the pan and set them aside. Stir-fry the snow peas for an additional three minutes after they've been added to the pan. Add the soy sauce mixture, bring to a boil, and keep stirring. Slowly bring down the heat and allow the sauce to simmer until it reaches the desired consistency. Serve at once.

TENDER BAKED CHICKEN IN ITALY.

4 To sum it up, the prep time is 10 minutes and the cooking time is 20. There are 55.9 calories, 17.1 grams of carbohydrates and 31.8 grams of protein in this meal.

When it comes to the ingredients, you'll need: 3 cups of mayonnaise, 3 cups of breadcrumbs (Italian-seasoned), and 2 cups of grated Parmesan cheese. DIRECTIONS

Set the temperature of the oven to 425 degrees Fahrenheit before beginning.

Garlic powder, mayonnaise, and Parmesan cheese should be mixed together in a bowl before serving. In a separate bowl, combine the bread crumbs and water.

bowl. To coat the chicken, first dip it in the mayonnaise mixture and then in the bread crumbs. Place the chicken in a single layer on a baking sheet.

Bake for 20 minutes, or until the chicken juices run clear and the coating is golden brown, in a preheated oven at 350 degrees Fahrenheit.

BOSTON BAKED BEANS

Servings: Six - Prep: 30m - Cooks: 4h - Total: 5h - Additional: 30m A FEW FACTS ABOUT DIET There are 382 calories in this serving, with 63.1 grams of carbohydrates, 6.3 grams of fat, 20.7 grams of protein, and 14 milligrams of cholesterol. INGREDIENTS: 2 cups navy beans, 1/4 teaspoon black pepper, 1/2 pound bacon, 1/4 teaspoon dry mustard, 1 finely diced onion, 1/2 cup ketchup, 3 tablespoons molasses, 1 tablespoon Worcestershire sauce, 2 teaspoons salt, 1/4 cup brown sugar.

Prepare beans by soaking in cold water overnight. For about 1 to 1 1/2 hours, simmer the beans until they are soft but not falling apart.

Two and a half hours. Reserve the liquid by draining it.

Set the oven temperature to 325 degrees F.

Place a portion of the beans at the bottom of a 2-quart bean pot or casserole dish.

Bacon and onion are then layered on top of the pasta in the dish

molasses salt pepper dry mustard ketchup Worcestershire sauce brown sugar brown sugar in a saucepan. Stir in beans after the mixture has come to a boil. The beans should be completely covered by the remaining bean water. A lid or aluminum foil can be used to protect the food from the elements.

In a preheated oven, cook the beans for 3 to 4 hours or until they are tender. In order to prevent the beans from becoming too dry, remove the lid about halfway through the cooking process.

SPINACH WITH A CHIPOTLE CRUSS CRUST

Servings: Six - Preparation: 15m - Cooking: 20m - Total: 35m - A FEW FACTS ABOUT DIET

183 calories, 11.7 grams of carbohydrate, 6.1 grams of fat, 20.4 grams of protein, and 62 milligrams of cholesterol are the nutritional stats for this dish.

The following ingredients are used in this recipe: 1 tbsp. onion powder, 1 1/2 tsp. salt, 1 tbsp. garlic powder, 4 tbsp. brown sugar, 3 tbsp. chipotle chile powder, and 2 (3/4 pounds) loin chops, sliced thinly

Grill on medium-high heat for a few minutes.

Use a large resealable plastic bag to combine the chipotle chile and salt with the onion and garlic powders. Tenderloins should be placed in a bag and shook to evenly coat the meat. Refrigerate for ten to fifteen minutes before using the recipe.

Grill the meat on a lightly oiled grill grate. Cook the meat for 20 minutes, flipping it over every 5 minutes or so.. Slice after 5 to 10 minutes of resting on the grill.

PANCAKES

How many servings are there? - Prep: 5m - Cooks: 10m - Total: 20m - CARBOHYDRATES 40.2g; Fat 13g; Protein 9g; Cholesterol 69 mg per serving in NUTRITION FACTS

INGREDIENTS

In a bowl, combine the following ingredients: 1 cup all-purpose flour, 1/4 teaspoon salt, 1/2 teaspoon baking soda, 1 tablespoon white sugar, 1 cup milk, 1 teaspoon baking powder, 1 egg, and 2 tablespoons of vegetable oil.
DIRECTIONS

Pre-heat a medium-high griddle with a little oil. Watch Now!

Baking soda and baking powder can be added to the flour mixture. Create a well in the middle of the table. Separate from this

Egg, milk, and oil are mixed in a bowl. Pour the milk mixture into the flour mixture and mix thoroughly. To achieve a silky finish, add all of the ingredients to

Watch Now!

To begin, pour or scoop a quarter cup of batter onto the griddle. Serve immediately after browning both sides. Click here to see it now.

POLLO FAJITAS

Servings per recipe: 5 Additional: 30m - Prep: 15m Cooks: 10m - Total: 55m A FEW FACTS ABOUT DIET

Protein: 27.6; Carbohydrate: 5.8; Cholesterol: 113mg; Total: 209.7 Calories;

In order to make this dish, you'll need 1 tablespoon Worcestershire sauce, 1 1/2 pounds of boneless, skinless chicken thighs, a cup of cider vinegar, a tablespoon of vegetable oil, a tablespoon of soy sauce, a clove of garlic, minced and a dash of hot pepper sauce.

DIRECTIONS

Combine Worcestershire sauce, vinegar, soy sauce, chili powder, garlic, and a dash of heat in a medium bowl.

Sauce with a kick of heat. Turn the chicken once in the sauce to ensure that it is well-coated. Prepare the marinade for 30 minutes at room temperature, or overnight in the refrigerator.

Using a large skillet set over high heat, warm oil. Sauté the chicken strips for five minutes after they've been added to the pan. Continue to cook for an additional 3 minutes after adding the onion and green pepper. Serve with lemon juice on the side.

Sarah's Pilaf of Rice

4 Preparation: 10m - Cooking: 35m - Total: 50m - Additional: 5m Nutrition Facts: 244 calories, 40 grams of carbohydrates, 6.5 grams of fat, 5.9 grams of protein, and 18 milligrams of cholesterol. orzo pasta, 1/2 cup uncooked white rice, and 1/2 cup chopped onion f 2 cups chicken broth f 2 tbsp. butter f 2 cloves of minced garlic Over medium-low heat, melt the butter in a covered skillet. Cook and stir the orzo pasta until it is golden brown.

Then add the onion and cook until it is translucent, followed by the garlic and cooking for an additional 30-seconds. Be sure to incorporate all ingredients before serving. Bring to a rolling boil over high heat. Once rice is tender and liquid has been absorbed, turn heat down to medium-low and cover to simmer for 20 to 25 minutes. Fluff with a fork after removing from the heat for 5 minutes.

BACK-TO-OUR-ORIGIN PANCAKES

4 - Preparation: 5m - Cooking: 20m - Total: 25m - Three hundred and one eighty-nine 43.7g of carbohydrates, 11.9g of fat, and 9g of protein. 75 milligrams of cholesterol

FILLINGS f 1 1/2 cups all-purpose flour 1 1/2 cups baking powder 1 egg 1 teaspoon salt 1 1/4 cups milk 1 tablespoon white sugar cooking spray 3 1/2 teaspoons baking powder

DIRECTIONS

Using a whisk or fork, combine the dry ingredients in a large mixing bowl.

Add the melted butter, egg, and milk, and whisk until well-combined and smooth. Allow the batter to rest for five minutes before serving. 3. Heat a large skillet to medium-high heat. Cooking spray should be used. Pour the batter into the already-heated pan, and

approximately one-quarter cup of batter per pancake Each pancake should be cooked for 2 to 3 minutes, until bubbles appear on the sides and center. Flip and cook for an additional 1 to 2 minutes or until golden.

RICE CASSEROLE WITH CHICKEN AND BROCCOLI AND RICE BROCCOLI

Tablespoons: Eight - Preparation: 15m - Cooking: 30m - Total: 45m - There are 756 calories, 82.7 grams of carbohydrates and 36 grams of protein in this meal. There is 109.5 milligrams of cholesterol in this meal.

ingredients: 2 cups water, 1/4 cup melted butter, 2 cups instant rice, 1 cup milk, two 10-ounce cans of chunk chicken, drained, one 16-ounce package of frozen chopped broccoli, one 10-ounce can of condensed cream of mushroom soup, one small chopped white onion, one 10-ounce can of condensed cream of chicken soup, and one pound of processed cheese food

DIRECTIONS

350 degrees Fahrenheit is the ideal temperature for baking

Boil the water in a medium saucepan. Then add the instant rice and cover the pot.

Allow for five minutes of rest.

Prepare the rice, chicken, mushroom soup, chicken soup, butter, milk, broccoli, onion, and processed cheese in a 9-by-13-inch baking dish.

Bake for 30 to 35 minutes, or until the cheese is melted, in a preheated oven. Halfway through cooking, stir to ensure even melting of the cheese.

Burgers in the style of mini sliders.

Servings per recipe: twenty-four Cooks: 40 minutes; 10 minutes for prep; 50 minutes total. A FEW FACTS ABOUT DIET

232 calories, 16.1 grams of carbohydrates, 13.2 grams of fat, 12 grams of protein, and 36 milligrams of cholesterol.

This recipe calls for two pounds of ground beef, two cups of chopped Cheddar cheese, and one (1.25-ounce) envelope of onion soup mix.

2 cups mayonnaise f 2 cups chopped pickle slices

WHERE TO START Pre-heat the oven to 350°F Spritz a baking sheet with cooking spray before placing aluminum foil on top of it.

with cooking spray

In a large skillet, combine the ground beef and the onion soup mix and cook, stirring frequently, until the beef is crumbly, evenly browned, and no longer pink in the middle. Excess grease should be drained and thrown away.

Removing the food from the heat is necessary. Stir in the mayonnaise and Cheddar cheese to the meat mix before dishing out to guests. 3) Place the dinner rolls' undersides on the baking sheet that has been prepared. Top each roll with a half-and-half mixture of cheese and ground beef. Reinstall the aprons. Spray a second sheet of aluminum foil with cooking spray before placing it on top.

4. Cook for 30 minutes in a preheated oven until the burgers are hot and the cheese is melted. Pickles, sliced, should be served on the side.

Chips made with boiled potatoes

Servings: four. - 30 minutes for preparation - 5 minutes for cooking - 35 minutes total Nutrient Facts: 80 calories, 11.6 grams of carbohydrates, 3.5 grams of fat, 1.2 grams of protein, 0 milligrams of cholesterol

TOTAL INGREDIENTS: 1 tablespoon of vegetable oil, 1 medium potato, thinly sliced (peel optional) A pinch of salt, or to your liking. DIRECTIONS

The vegetable oil should be placed in a plastic bag (a produce bag works well). Shake the potato pieces into the mixture.

coat.

Apply a little coating of oil or frying spray on a large dinner dish. Place the sliced potatoes in a single layer in the serving dish.

3 to 5 minutes in the microwave should do the trick, or until they've browned a little. The cooking time will be affected by the microwave's power. Take the chips off the dish and season with salt (or other seasonings). Let it cool down a little. It's time to do it all over again! No more re-oiling of the plate.

Chapter Four

AWESOME GREEN BEANS CASSEROLE

How many portions are there? Preparation: 10m - Cooking: 15m - Total: 25m FACTS ABOUT DIET AND FITNESS

20.2g of carbs, 23.2g of fat, 6.6g of protein, and 20mg of cholesterol make up this meal's total caloric content.

This recipe calls for 2 cans of green beans that have been drained, along with 1 can of condensed cream of mushroom soup and a cup of Cheddar cheese, all of which can be found in the pantry.

DIRECTIONS

Make sure the oven is preheated to 350 degrees Fahrenheit (175 degrees C).

Then, microwave the green beans and the soup in a big, microwave-safe bowl. Stir well and warm in a microwave oven set to high.

until the temperature reaches a comfortable level (3 to 5 minutes). Reheat the mixture, adding the remaining 1/2 cup of cheese, for an additional 2 to 3 minutes. Transfer the green bean mixture to a casserole dish and top it with French fried onions and the remaining cheese.

Bake at 175 degrees Celsius (175 degrees Fahrenheit) until the cheese is melted and the onions are beginning to brown, about 10 minutes.

FAST AND EASY CHICKEN FROM AIMEE

Servings: four. - 5 minutes for preparation, 30 minutes for cooking, a total of 35 minutes. Nutrient Facts: 242.5 calories, 8.8 grams of carbohydrates, 32.4 grams of protein, and 81 milligrams of cholesterol. Skinless, boneless breast halves of 4 chicken breasts each, 1/4 cup bacon bits and 4oz. water Half a cup of grated Parmesan cheese and 1/4 cup of teriyaki sauce go well together in this dish. DIRECTIONS

The oven should be preheated at 400 degrees Fahrenheit (200 degrees C).

The dish should be 9x13 inches in size. Place chicken in a large serving dish, add mustard, and then teriyaki sauce to taste.

evenly distributed. Bacon bits should be sprinkled on top, followed by cheese.

30-minute baking time at a temperature of 400°F (200°C).

QUICHE IS EASY TO MAKE.

Tablespoons: Eight It takes 10 minutes to prep, and another 50 minutes to cook.

Eating a diet high in fat and cholesterol can raise your risk for heart disease.

There are four eggs and two cups of milk in this recipe.

1 package (about 10 ounces) of thawed and drained chopped frozen broccoli F 8 ounces of shredded Cheddar cheese f 1/4 cup of softened butter

DIRECTIONS

Start by preheating the oven to 375°F (190 degrees C). A 10-inch quiche pan should be lightly greased. A large bowl should be filled with milk, eggs and baking mix, as well as the butter and parmesan cheese. 2. Lumps are expected in the batter.

Add broccoli, ham, and Cheddar cheese to the mixture. Pour into the prepared quiche dish.

To bake, place the dish in a preheated oven and bake for 50 minutes, or until the eggs are set and the top is browned.

Honey Pecan Pork Chops are delicious.

Servings: four. - 15 minutes for preparation, 10 minutes for cooking, a total of 25 minutes. COMPLETE NUTRITION

INFORMATION Percent Daily Values (DV): Cholesterol: 100mg, Fat: 30.7g, Protein 30.6g, Carbohydrates: 30.3.

1/4 cup honey, salt, and pepper to taste, 1 1/4 pounds pounded thin boneless pork loin, 2 tablespoons butter, 1/2 cup all-purpose flour for coating, and 1/4 cup chopped pecans DIRECTIONS

Combine the flour, salt, and pepper in a large bowl. Dip pork cutlets in the flour mixture and then fry them.

Over medium-high heat, melt the butter in a large skillet. Brown both sides of the chops by adding them to the pan.

Make the switch to a new

Warm food.

Add honey and pecans to the drippings from the skillet. Stirring constantly, bring to a boil. Cutlets should be drenched in the sauce.

SOUPE A L'AVOCADO DE NACHO

How many portions are there? - Preparation: 15m - Cooking: 20m - Total: 35m - FACTS ABOUT DIET AND FITNESS

Calories: 497; carbohydrates: 23.9g; fats: 33.6g; proteins: 26.1g; and cholesterol: 98 milligrams;

3 tablespoons creamy salad dressing 2 cups Colby cheese 2 cups whole kernel corn drained 2 cups shredded tortilla chips

f 1 tablespoon chili powder 2 cups crushed tortilla chips f 1 (10 ounce) can of whole kernel corn (e.g. Miracle Whip)

DIRECTIONS

The oven should be preheated to 350 degrees Fahrenheit (175 degrees C).

Stir-fry ground beef in a medium-sized skillet. Cook until evenly distributed, stirring frequently to prevent sticking.

browned. Drain the grease from your pans. Immediately after removing it from the heat, stir in the salsa and chili powder. Layer the ground beef, tortilla chips, and cheese twice in a 2-quart casserole dish, finishing with cheese on top.

The dish should be thoroughly warmed and the cheese should be completely melted, about 20 minutes in an oven preheated to 350 degrees Fahrenheit.

THE SEASONING FOR FAJITA

Servings: four. Preparation: 5m - Cooks: 0m - Total: 5m FACTS ABOUT DIET AND FITNESS

21, Carbohydrates 4.6g Fat 0,4g Protein 0,4g Cholesterol 0mg Calories 21

1/2 teaspoon onion powder, 1/2 teaspoon chili powder, 1/2 teaspoon garlic powder, and 1/4 teaspoon cayenne pepper are just some of the spices you'll need to make this dish. INSTRUCTIONS: 1. In a large bowl, whisk together the cornstarch and the remaining ingredients.

combine the cumin and salt in a small bowl.

CHICKEN, GREEN BEANS AND CHERRY TOMATOES

How many portions are there? - Preparation: 5m - Cooking: 15m - Total: 20m FACTS ABOUT DIET AND FITNESS

Calories 122, Carbohydrates 12.6g, Fat 8g, Protein 2.6g, Cholesterol 20mg.

2 cups trimmed and thinly sliced green beans 1 1/2 pounds 1/2 cup water, 3/4 teaspoon garlic salt, 1/4 teaspoon pepper, 1 1/2 tablespoons chopped fresh basil, 1 tablespoon sugar, 2 cups cherry tomato halves, 1 tablespoon sugar, and 3/4 teaspoon garlic salt

DIRECTIONS

Add the beans and water to a large saucepan and bring to a simmer. Pour water in and bring to a boil. Simmer for 10 minutes on low heat, or until vegetables are tender. Remove water from drain and place aside.

Melt the butter in a medium skillet. Bring to a boil and then reduce heat to low. Cook, stirring occasionally, until softened, the tomatoes. Toss the green beans gently with the tomato mixture before serving.

Perfectly mashed potatoes.

Servings: four. - Prep: 20 minutes; Cooks: 20 minutes; Total: 40 minutes. FACTS ABOUT DIET AND FITNESS

Fat: 12.7 grams; carbohydrates: 49.7 grams; protein: 6.7 grams; and cholesterol: 34 milligrams per serving.

Ingredients: f 3 large russet potatoes, peeled and cut in half lengthwise, f 1/4 cup butter, and 1/2 cup whole milk

DIRECTIONS

In a large pot, cover the potatoes with salted water and cook for about 30 minutes. Boil the water, turn the heat down and simmer for about 20 to 25 minutes, or until the vegetables are fork-tender. Return the potatoes to the pot after draining. For about 30 seconds, raise the heat to medium-high and allow the potatoes to dry out. Turn off the thermostat.

Add the butter and milk after mashing the potatoes twice around the pot with a potato masher. Mash until fluffy and smooth, and then serve. About 15 seconds of whisking should be enough to distribute the salt and black pepper.

Savory Biscuits and Gravy for Sausage

Tablespoons: Eight - Prep: 5m - Cooks: 10m - Total: 15m - A 333-calorie diet contains 30.8 grams of carbohydrates, 18.7 grams of fat, and 9.8 grams of protein, with a cholesterol content of 25 milligrams per serving.

Ingredients include a 16-ounce can of refrigerated jumbo buttermilk biscuits, 2 1/2 cups of milk, and a 9.6-ounce package of powdered milk powder. Original Pork Sausage Crumbles from Jimmy Dean f Flour with salt and pepper to taste f 1/4 cup

DIRECTIONS

To prepare the biscuits, follow the manufacturer's instructions on the packaging.

Cook sausage for 5-6 minutes, or until thoroughly heated, in a large skillet.

agitating the pot a few times a day. Add flour to the mixture. Stirring constantly, bring the mixture to a boil and thicken it. Two minutes later, turn the heat down to medium-low and continue to stir. Toss in some salt and pepper to taste.

Cookies should be halved before consuming them. Top each plate with a half-and-half and about a third of a cup of the gravy.

CORN SALSA SAUCE FOR FIREY FISH TACOS

How many portions are there? 30 minutes of preparation and 10 minutes of cooking equals a total of 40 minutes. calories 351, carbs 40,3, fat 9,6, protein 28,7 grams cholesterol 43 milligrams)

1 tablespoon ground black pepper 1 cup diced red onion
1 teaspoon salt, or to taste 2 teaspoons oil 1 cup fresh
cilantro leaves, chopped 12 warmed corn taco shells 1 lime,
juiced and zested 2 tablespoons sour cream, or to taste 2
tablespoons cayenne pepper, or to taste 3 cups cooked corn
kernels 5 teaspoon salt, or to taste 6 (4-ounce) fillets of tilapia
1 teaspoon salt, or to taste

Preheat the grill to high heat.

This dish can be made in advance and stored in the
refrigerator. Add the lime juice and mix well. Add salt and
pepper to taste.

and a dash of zing.

Add cayenne pepper, ground black pepper, and salt to a small
bowl and mix thoroughly.

Spices to taste should be sprinkled over each fillet after it has
been brushed with olive oil.

Grill the fillets for 3 minutes on each side, then remove them
from the grill. Two corn tortillas should be used to make each
fiery fish taco, with the fish, sour cream, and corn salsa placed
on top.

CASSEROLE WITH EGGS AND SAUSAGE.

The number of servings is 12 Prepare 15 minutes, cook
35 minutes and eat 50 mins Nutrition Facts: Calories: 341,

Carbohydrates: 8.7g, Fat: 24.7g, Protein: 19.9g, Cholesterol: 177mg

8 eggs, beaten, 1 teaspoon dried oregano, 2 cups shredded mozzarella cheese, 8 ounces refrigerated crescent roll dough, 2 cups shredded Cheddar cheese, and 1 teaspoon dried basil

DIRECTIONS

In a large skillet, cook the sausage. Cook until golden brown all over on a medium-high heat. Crumble and drain

put on the shelf

325 degrees Fahrenheit is the ideal temperature for baking (165 degrees C). A 9x13-inch baking dish should be lightly sprayed with cooking spray before use.

Crumbled sausage and crescent roll dough cover the bottom of the baking dish. Combine the beaten eggs, mozzarella, and Cheddar cheese in a large bowl and stir until well-combined. Oregano can be added to the mixture before it is poured over the sausage and rolls.

Bake for 25 to 30 minutes, or until a knife inserted in the center comes out clean, in a preheated oven.

CABBAGE FRIED TO PERfection

Servings: six. The total cooking time is 45 minutes: 20 minutes for prepping, 25 minutes for cooking, and 10 minutes for cleanup. CALORIES AND NUTRIENTS: 47, Cholesterol: 5 mg, Fat: 2g, Protein: 2.8g, Carbohydrates: 5.2g

1 teaspoon white sugar 1/4 cup minced onion 1/4 cup salt and pepper to taste 6 cups shaved cabbage 1 tablespoon vinegar 2 tablespoons water INGREDIENTS DIRECTIONS Heat a large, deep pan over medium-high heat and add the bacon. Cook until uniformly browned on both sides over medium-high heat. Cut out the bacon.

and then put away.

When the onion is soft, remove it from the bacon oil and set it aside. Add the cabbage and season with pepper, salt, sugar, and water.

Cook for approximately 15 minutes, or until the cabbage has wilted. Mix with some bacon. Before serving, give everything a good squirt of vinegar.

PEPPER STEAK FROM CHINA

Servings: four The total cooking time is 30 minutes: FACTS ABOUT DIET AND HEALTH

312 calories, 17 grams of carbohydrates, 15.4 grams of fat, 26.1 grams of protein, 69 milligrams of cholesterol

1 pound top sirloin beef steak 3 tablespoons vegetable oil divided 1/4 cup soy sauce 1 red onion cut into 1-inch squares 2 tablespoons white sugar 1 green bell pepper cut into 1-inch

squares 2 tablespoons cornstarch 2 tomatoes cut into wedges 1/2 teaspoon ground ginger INGREDIENTS 1 pound top sirloin beef steak 3 tablespoons vegetable oil divided Slice the meat against the grain into 1/2-inch thick pieces.

The sugar and cornstarch must be completely dissolved before adding the ginger and soy sauce to a bowl.

Smoothness is seen in the blend. Stir the marinade thoroughly before adding the steak pieces. In a wok or big pan, heat 1 tablespoon of vegetable oil over medium-high heat and add 1/3 of the steak strips. Remove the meat from the pan and set it aside in a bowl until it has browned, approximately 3 minutes. Cook the remaining beef in the same manner for a total of three more times, then put aside the cooked meat.

Return the meat to the pan, along with the onion, and cook until the onion is translucent. Stir in the green pepper after the meat and onion have been cooking for approximately 2 minutes. About 2 minutes after adding the peppers and stirring everything together, the tomatoes may be added. Once everything has been well mixed together, it's time to serve!

The ORECCHIETTE PASTA IS IN ONE PAN

How many people will be served? Preparation: 15m - Cooking: 25m - Total: 40m It has 662 calories, 46.2 grams of carbs and

39.1 grams of fat, 31.2 grams of protein, and 60 milligrammes of cholesterol.

1 1/4 cups orecchiette pasta or more to taste f salt to taste f half a cup coarsely chopped arugula, or to taste f 2 tablespoons olive oil f 3 1/2 cups low-sodium chicken broth

1/4 cup coarsely grated Parmigiano-Reggiano cheese or to taste f 8 ounces spicy Italian sausages, casings removed f

DIRECTIONS: In a large, deep pan, heat the olive oil over medium heat until shimmering but not smoking. Sauté the onion in a little olive oil with a sprinkle of salt until translucent.

5 to 7 minutes to soften and golden-brown the onion in the oil. Cook and stir sausage and onions for 5 to 7 minutes, or until the sausage is browned and crumbled.

Using a wooden spoon, scrape the brown pieces of food from the bottom of the pan while you heat 1 1/2 cups of chicken stock into sausage mixture. Toss orecchiette pasta into a pot of boiling water; simmer and stir for approximately 15 minutes until pasta is done and most of the stock is absorbed.

While spaghetti and sausages are cooking, add the arugula and stir until it is wilted. Dip the spaghetti with Parmigiano Reggiano cheese before serving it to your guests.

Burgers from CHRIS' BAY AREA

Servings: four - 10 minutes for preparation, 20 minutes for cooking, a total of 30 minutes. FACTS ABOUT DIET AND HEALTH

393 calories, 22.6 grams of carbohydrate, 22.6 grams of fat, 22.9 grams of protein, and 71 milligrams of cholesterol.

GRAIN BROWN BEEF: 2 cloves minced garlic, 1 teaspoon freshly ground black pepper, 1/2 teaspoon dried basil, 2 tablespoons extra virgin olive oil, 4 split hamburger buns, 1 1/2 teaspoon salt. DIRECTIONS

Prepare a gas or charcoal grill for high temperatures. Combine the meat, garlic, olive oil, salt, and pepper in a large bowl.

basil. Flatten into patties after being divided into four equal halves.

For medium-rare or well-done results, cook the patties for 3 to 5 minutes on each side. A minimum internal temperature of 160 degrees Fahrenheit is required (70 degrees C). Hamburger buns are ready when the meat is taken off of the grill. Add favorite condiments and garnishes before serving.

CHICKEN BURRITO FUEL WITH SALSA SAUCE

Servings: four - 5 minutes of prep time, 30 minutes of cooking time, and a final time investment of 35 minutes. CALORIES, PROTEIN, AND CHOLESTEROL IN THIS MEAL: 107.1, 9.6, 12.3, and 30.4 milligrams per serving

This recipe calls for the following ingredients: f 2 skinless, boneless chicken breast halves 2 tablespoons ground cumin 1 tablespoon ground chili powder 1 tablespoon taco seasoning mix 2 cloves chopped garlic 1/4 cup salsa 1 teaspoon chili powder

In a medium saucepan, cook the tomato sauce and the chicken breasts over medium-high heat. Bring to a boil

then add the salsa, seasoning, cumin, garlic, and chili powder. Let it cook for 15 minutes. 2. Start separating the chicken flesh into thin strands with a fork. Cook the pulled chicken flesh and sauce for another 5 to 10 minutes, covered, until the meat is tender. Stir in the spicy sauce to taste. (Note: If the mixture thickens too much due to being cooked at a high temperature, you may need to add a little water.)

ORZO NOODLES WITH GARLIC CHICKEN

Servings: four The total cooking time is 30 minutes: There are 350.7 calories, 40.4 grams of carbohydrate, 22 grams of protein, and 38.1 milligrams of cholesterol in this serving.

2 tablespoons olive oil 1 tablespoon finely chopped fresh parsley 2 cloves minced garlic 2 cups fresh spinach leaves 1/4 teaspoon crushed red pepper 2 tablespoons grated Parmesan cheese for garnishing INGREDIENTS 1 cup uncooked orzo pasta 1/8 teaspoon salt to taste Bite-sized chicken breast halves from two skinless and boneless chicken breast halves

DIRECTIONS

To begin, bring a big pot of lightly salted water to a boil over high heat. Orzo pasta should be al dente after 8 to 10 minutes of cooking.

draining and dente.

Cook the garlic and red pepper for one minute in a pan over medium-high heat, until the garlic is golden brown. Cook for 2 to 5 minutes, until the chicken is gently browned and the juices flow clear, then add salt to taste. Toss in the cooked orzo and parsley, and lower the heat. In a large pan, cook the spinach until it is just wilted. Stirring regularly, cook for a further 5 minutes or until spinach has wilted. Serve with more Parmesan on top.

Chapter Five

CHIPS OF HERBED PORK

Servings: four - Preparation: 10m - Cooking: 25m - Total: 35m - FACTS ABOUT DIET AND HEALTH

This meal has 601 calories, 10.9 grams of carbohydrates, 43.6 grams of fat, 40 grams of protein, and 165 milligrams of cholesterol per serving.

This recipe calls for four thick-cut pork chops, one teaspoon of Montreal steak seasoning, and one tablespoon of dried basil. It also calls for one teaspoon of instant beef bouillon, half a cup of butter, and two tablespoons of all-purpose flour, as well as two cups of milk.

Pork chops should be seasoned with Montreal steak seasoning on both sides.

Over medium heat, melt 2 tablespoons of butter in a large pan. Chops should be cooked in melted butter before being served.

Cooking time should be between seven and ten minutes each side. Insert an instant-read thermometer into the middle and it should register at least 145 degrees F. (63 degrees C). When the chops are done cooking, remove approximately 3 tablespoons of pan drippings from the pan and add the remaining butter. Return the skillet to a medium-high heat and add the pork chops.

In a bowl, combine flour, basil, and beef bouillon. Cook for one minute with the pan drippings and black pepper in a skillet. Continue to whisk regularly for approximately 2 minutes after putting in the flour mixture and cooking for another minute. Cook and stir regularly until the mixture is thick and bubbling, 4 to 6 minutes after adding the milk to the flour mixture. Serve the pork chops with the sauce.

The Sauce Is Sweet and Sour

Dozens of meals: Cooks: 10m, Prep: 2m, Total: 12m CALORIES: 43; CARBOS: 10.8; FATS: 0; PROTEINS: 0.3; CHOLESTEROL: 0

1 tablespoon ketchup 1 1/3 cups water 2 teaspoons cornstarch 1 3/4 cups white sugar 1/4 cup soy sauce 1/3 cups white vinegar 1 tablespoon ketchup 1 1/3 cups water

HOW TO MAKE 1. In a medium-sized saucepan over medium-high heat combine the sugar, vinegar, water, soy sauce, ketchup, and cornstarch and bring to a boil.

boil. Stir the mixture constantly until it has thickened, about 5 minutes.

Simple Beef Stroganoff Recipe

Servings: four - 20 minutes for preparation, 10 minutes for cooking, a total of 30 minutes. FACTS ABOUT DIET AND HEALTH

679 calories, 48.2 grams of carbs, 40.5 grams of fat, 28.7 grams of protein, and 159 milligrams of cholesterol.

Ingredients include 1 (8 ounce) package of egg noodles, 1 tablespoon of garlic powder, a pound of mince beef, and 1/2 cup of sour cream. Salt and pepper to taste are also included.

DIRECTIONS

Set aside the egg noodles once they have been prepared in accordance with the package guidelines.

Over medium heat, cook ground beef for 5 to 10 minutes in a separate large pan

cook for a few minutes, or until golden brown. Add the soup and garlic powder when the fat has been drained. Ten minutes into the simmering process, stir periodically.

Serve with a side of egg noodles and the meat mixture. Salt and pepper to taste before adding the sour cream.

BEANS THAT ARE BOTH SALTY AND SWEET.

Servings: four Cooks: 10 minutes; 15 minutes for preparation; 25 minutes total. FACTS ABOUT DIET AND HEALTH

Carbohydrates: 8.6g; Fat: 2.4g; Protein: 2.1g; Cholesterol: 0mg; 59 calories.

INGREDIENTS

2 tablespoons canola oil 2 cloves minced garlic 14 cup fresh green beans, trimmed 2 tablespoons soy sauce 14 teaspoon honey 14 cup minced garlic DIRECTIONS

Steam the green beans for 3 to 4 minutes in a steamer basket placed in a saucepan of boiling water. Add the honey, soy sauce, garlic, and chili sauce to a mixing bowl.

3. In a medium-sized skillet, warm the canola oil. Toss in the green beans, and cook for 3 to 5 minutes. Pour

dissolved in the soy sauce. The liquid should be almost completely evaporated after another 2 minutes of boiling and stirring. Serve right away.

WEST ITALIAN CASEROLE PASTA

Servings: Eight It took 45 minutes to cook and 15 minutes to prep. calories 380, carbs 32, fat 21, protein 16, cholesterol 23, fat 21, protein 16, protein 16, cholesterol 23, dietary cholesterol 23

1 uncooked 8-ounce box of penne pasta, 1/2 teaspoon dried basil, 2 tablespoons olive oil, 2 cups milk, 1/2 pound thinly

sliced portobellos, 2 cups shredded mozzarella cheese, 1/2 cup margarine, 1 cup sour cream, 1 cup parmesan cheese, 1 cup sour cream, 1 cup parmesan cheese (10 ounce) 1/4 cup all-purpose flour 1/4 cup soy sauce and 1 big bulb minced garlic in the bag of frozen chopped spinach

DIRECTIONS

Pre-heat the oven to 350 degrees Fahrenheit (175 degrees Celsius) (175 degrees C). A 9x13-inch baking dish should be lightly greased. Then bring up to a rolling boil a big saucepan of liberally salted water. Cook the pasta for 8 to 10 minutes, or until al dente.

draining and dente.

3. In a medium-sized saucepan, warm the oil. Add the mushrooms, cook for a minute, then remove from the heat. In a saucepan, heat the margarine until it's melted. Gather all the ingredients and begin to combine them. Add milk one tablespoon at a time, mixing well after each addition. Toss in 1 cup of the cheese and heat through. Toss cooked pasta, mushrooms, spinach, and soy sauce together in the pot. Top with the remaining cheese and bake as directed. For the last step, bake for 20 minutes in a preheated oven.

FRESHLY BAKED CARROTS

Servings: four. - 10 minutes for preparation, 30 minutes for cooking, a total of 40 minutes. Facts Calories 150, Carbs 24.5g, Fat 6g, Protein 1.22g, Cholesterol 15mg. Nutrition Facts

To make 1 pound of diced carrots, mix together 1 teaspoon salt, 2 tablespoons of diced butter, 1 pinch of ground black pepper, and 1/4 cup of packed brown sugar. Place the carrots in a pot filled with salted water. Once you've brought the water to a rolling boil, lower the heat to a gentle simmer, and cook for about

Approximately 20 to 30 minutes. Don't overcook the carrots to the point of being mushy!

Re-add the carrots to the pan after draining and lowering the heat to its lowest setting possible. Add salt and pepper to taste, along with the butter and brown sugar. When the sugar has dissolved and is bubbling, the mixture is done cooking. Serve at once.

CHICKEN WINGS, BAKED IN THE OVEN

Tablespoons: Two - Preparation: 10m - Cooking: 1h - Total: 1h10m - It has 532.1 calories, 3.9 grams of carbohydrate, 31 grams of protein, and 96.6 milligrams of cholesterol.

INGREDIENTS

3 tbsp. of extra virgin olive oil

garlic powder, 1 tsp.

Pressed garlic from three cloves

As much salt and pepper as you like.

2 tbsp. chili powder.

10 pieces of chicken wing chicken

DIRECTIONS

The oven should be preheated to 375 degrees F. (190 degrees C).

A large, resealable bag should be used to combine the olive oil and garlic, as well as salt and pepper.

To combine, place the seal in an airtight container and give it a good shake Shake the container before adding the chicken wings. Bake the chicken wings in a single layer on a baking pan.

Cook the wings in a preheated oven for one hour or until they are crispy and cooked through.

PORK CHOP SALAD WITH CARAMELIZED ONION CARAMELIZATION

Servings: four. - 5 minutes for preparation, 40 minutes for cooking, a total of 45 minutes. Nutrition Facts: Calories: 47, Carbohydrates: 4g, Fat: 3.5g, Protein: 0.5g, Cholesterol: 0mg.

FOUR (4-ounce) pork loin chops (half-inch thick), seasoned with three teaspoons of salt, one onion (cut into thin strips), and one cup of water are the only ingredients needed to make this dish. DIRECTIONS

2 tsp. salt and 1 tsp. pepper, or to taste, should be applied to the chops before cooking.

Heat oil in a frying pan over medium heat. Pork chops should be browned on both sides. In a large bowl, mix together the onions, water, and salt.

pan. Simmer covered for 20 minutes at a lower temperature.

Add the remaining salt and pepper to the chops after turning them over. Once water has evaporated and the onions have turned from light to medium brown, cover the pot and continue cooking. To serve, remove chops from the pan and top with onions.

Casarelo Tater Tot Taco

Tablespoons: Eight Total time: 1 hour and 15 minutes for preparation, 1 hour and 15 minutes for cooking. Nutrition Facts: Calories: 477, Carbohydrates: 38.4g, Fat: 27g, Protein: 24.9g, Cholesterol: 76mg, per serving

1 pound ground beef 1 can rinsed and drained 12 ounce can of black beans 1 small onion diced 12 ounce bag of Mexican cheese blend shredded 16 ounce bag of frozen tater tots 1 ounce packet of taco seasoning mix 1 pound ground beef F

1 enchilada sauce can and 1 (16 ounce) bag of Mexican-style corn frozen in the freezer

DIRECTIONS

The oven should be preheated to 375 degrees F. (190 degrees C). spray with cooking oil a 9 x 13-inch baking dish 2. In a skillet, brown the ground beef for 5 to 7 minutes on medium heat. Then, add the

After 10 minutes of cooking and stirring, add the ground beef with onion, garlic, taco seasoning, frozen Mexican-style corn, and black beans. Set aside for a few minutes to allow the heat to dissipate.

In a large bowl, mix the ground beef mixture with about 3/4 of the Mexican cheese blend and the tater tots.

Prepare the baking dish by laying down about 1/3 of the enchilada sauce. Pour in the tater tot mixture and pat it down into a single, even layer in the baking dish before baking. Over the tater tots, drizzle the remainder of the enchilada sauce over the entire dish.

Pre-heat the oven to 400 degrees Fahrenheit. Return the casserole to the oven and top with the remaining Mexican cheese until the cheese is melted and bubbly, about 5 minutes.

EITHER FOR YOUR FRIENDS OR A CROWD.

Servings: four. - Preparation: 5m - Cooking: 15m - Total: 20m

FACTS ABOUT DIET AND FITNESS

Foods with less than one-tenth as many calories as the recommended daily allowance (DV) as well as the following macronutrient composition:

INGREDIENTS

1 pound of thinly sliced bacon

Make sure the oven is preheated to 350 degrees Fahrenheit (175 degrees C). Alu-foil a baking sheet and set it aside. Bacon should be arranged on a baking sheet in a single layer, with the edges touching or slightly overlapping, so that they cook evenly.

Bake in a preheated oven for 10 to 15 minutes, depending on the desired doneness. Using tongs or a fork, remove bacon from the baking sheet and place on a paper towel-lined plate to drain.

Crab and Kielbasa

How many portions are there? - 10 minutes for preparation, 30 minutes for cooking, a total of 40 minutes. Calories: 377, Carbohydrates: 20.2g, Fat: 26g, Protein: 17.2g, Cholesterol: 63mg Nutrition Facts

INGREDIENTS

Bacon rashers of six

Red pepper flakes in a quarter teaspoon

a quarter cup of water and a quarter teaspoon of seasoning salt

2 tbsp. sugar, white

Caraway seed is 3 teaspoons.

Cabbage cut into small wedges and chopped onion

Garlic minced into 2 tablespoons

1 pound of Polish kielbasa

Fry the bacon in a medium-sized skillet over medium-high heat, turning once, until it's browned and crispy on all sides. Taking the bacon out of the dish

Placing it on paper towels will help absorb any excess grease.

Melt butter in a large saucepan over medium heat. Add water until a syrup forms. Add salt and caraway seeds at this point. Gentle stir in the cabbage. Cover and cook for 10 to 15 minutes on medium-high heat.

Make kielbasa in the pan. Cover and cook for another 10 to 15 minutes. Serve immediately with additional crumbled bacon.

CASSEROLE OF GREEN BEANS BY CAMPBELL

The number of servings is 12 - 10 minutes for preparation, 30 minutes for cooking, a total of 40 minutes. (2) 10.75-ounce cans of condensed mushroom soup or condensed 98 percent soup from Campbell's

1/4 teaspoon ground black pepper 1 cup milk 8 cups of cooked cut green beans 2 2/3 tablespoons soy sauce fried onions in the style of the French

DIRECTIONS

Serve with a side of steamed rice and garnished with a few slices of scallions.

At 350 degrees F, bake the dish for 25 minutes, or until it's heated through. Stir.

Sprinkle the rest of the onions on top. Bake another 5 minutes.

Cubes of Barbecued Beef

How many portions are there? - Preparation: 15m - Cooking: 25m - Total: 40m FACTS ABOUT DIET AND FITNESS

Carbohydrates: 32.4g, Fat: 17.2g, Protein: 16.5g, Cholesterol: 46mg.

2 pounds of lean ground beef, 1 package of chilled biscuit dough, 1/2 cup barbecue sauce, and 1/3 cup shredded Cheddar cheese are all that's needed to make this delicious sandwich.. DIRECTIONS

Make sure the oven is preheated to 350 degrees Fahrenheit (175 degrees C). Apply a thin layer of cooking spray to each muffin cup.

Cook the beef until it is well-browned and no longer pink in a large heavy skillet set over medium heat. Get rid of the extra fat. Add to the mix by whisking together.

The combination of barbeque sauce and dried onion is delicious. A few minutes of simmering are all that is needed.

Press each biscuit into the prepared muffin cups by flattening it out. Make sure that the dough reaches the top of the pan. Fill each dough cup halfway with the meat mixture and set aside.

For 12 minutes, preheat the oven to 350 degrees F. Add the cheese and bake for an additional three minutes.

A CAULIFLOWER WITH GARLIC MASH

Servings: four. - 15 minutes for preparation, 10 minutes for cooking, a total of 25 minutes. Nutrition Facts: 98 calories, 8.4 grams of carbohydrates, 5.7 grams of fat, 5.2 grams of protein, and 7 milligrams of cholesterol.

Components: 1/4 cup grated Parmesan cheese, 1/4 cup reduced-fat cream cheese, 1 clove crushed garlic, 1/2 teaspoon salt, 1/4 cup olive oil 1/8 tsp. black pepper, freshly ground

DIRECTIONS

Pour enough water into a saucepan to come halfway up the side of a steamer insert. Bring

bring a pot of water to a rolling boil. Cover and steam for about 10 minutes until the cauliflower is tender.

Cook and stir the garlic for 2 minutes in a small skillet of olive oil over medium heat. Removing the food from the heat is necessary.

Blend the cauliflower in a food processor until smooth. Cauliflower should be pureed to the desired consistency before being added. Using a mixer, combine the ingredients until smooth.

UGLIES

Tablespoons: Eight - 20 minutes for preparation, 15 minutes for cooking, a total of 40 minutes, plus an additional 5 minutes FACTS ABOUT DIET AND FITNESS Fat: 17.2g, Protein: 17g, Cholesterol: 56mg / 360 calories GROUND BEEF CHUCK: 1 pound grated beef chuck: 1 12 cups barbeque sauce: 1/2 cup minced onion: 1 package (10 ounces) chilled biscuit dough: half a teaspoon of garlic powder: 2 cups shredded Cheddar cheese

DIRECTIONS

Start by preheating the oven to 400°F (200 degrees C). Grease the tins of 8 muffin tins. Ground chuck, onion, and garlic powder should be cooked evenly in a large skillet or frying pan;

The grease should be removed. For an additional 3 minutes, add the barbeque sauce to the pot and continue to simmer. Using a floured surface, roll out each biscuit to a 6-inch diameter. A cup shape can be created by folding up both sides of an open biscuit into the muffin pan. Add the meat mixture to the biscuits, almost to the brim, and top with cheddar cheese.

4. Bake in preheated oven until biscuits are baked, cheese is melted and tops are golden brown, about 15\sminutes.

LIME CILANTRO RICE

Servings: four. Total preparation time is 30 minutes. FACTS ABOUT DIET AND FITNESS

Calories: 84, Carbohydrates: 12.7g, Fat: 3.1g, Protein: 2.4g, Cholesterol: 8mg

INGREDIENTS\sf 2 cups water\sf 1 teaspoon lime zest\sf 1 tablespoon butter\sf 2 tablespoons fresh lime juice\sf 1 cup long-grain white rice f 1/2 cup chopped cilantro DIRECTIONS

Bring the water to a boil; stir the butter and rice into the water. Cover, reduce heat to low, and simmer

until the rice is tender, about 20 minutes.

Stir the lime zest, lime juice, and cilantro into the cooked rice just before serving.

Chapter Six

ANDREA'S PASTA FAGIOLI

Tablespoons: Eight - Prep: 10m - Cooks: 1h30m - Total: 1h40m
NUTRITION FACTS\sCalories: 403, Carbohydrates: 68g, Fat: 7.6g, Protein: 16.3g, Cholesterol: 3mg

INGREDIENTS\sf 3 tablespoons olive oil\sf 1 1/2 teaspoons dried oregano f 1 onion, quartered then halved f 1 teaspoon salt\sf 2 cloves garlic, minced\sf 1 (15 ounce) can cannellini beans\sf 1 (29 ounce) can tomato sauce f 1 (15 ounce) can navy beans f 5 1/2 cups water\sf 1/3 cup grated Parmesan cheese\sf 1 tablespoon dried parsley\sf 1 pound ditalini pasta\sf 1 1/2 teaspoons dried basil

DIRECTIONS

In a large pot over medium heat, cook onion in olive oil until translucent. Stir in garlic and cook until tender. Reduce heat, and stir in tomato sauce, water, parsley, basil, oregano, salt, cannelini beans, navy beans and Parmesan. Simmer 1 hour.

Bring a big pot of water to a boil with a little salt in it. Add pasta and cook for 8 to 10 minutes or until al dente; drain. Stir into soup.

QUICK BAKED ZUCCHINI CHIPS

Servings: four. - Prep: 5m - Cooks: 10m - Total: 15m - FACTS ABOUT DIET AND FITNESS

Calories: 92, Carbohydrates: 13.8g, Fat: 1.7g, Protein: 6.1g, Cholesterol: 2mg

INGREDIENTS\sf 2 medium zucchini, cut into 1/4-inch slices\sf 2 tablespoons grated Parmesan cheese\sf 1/2 cup seasoned dry bread crumbs\sf 2 egg whites\sf 1/8 teaspoon ground black pepper

DIRECTIONS

Preheat the oven to 475 degrees F (245 degrees C) (245 degrees C).

In one small bowl, stir together the bread crumbs, pepper and Parmesan cheese. Place the egg whites in

a separate bowl. Dip zucchini slices into the egg whites, then coat the breadcrumb mixture. Place on a greased baking sheet.

Bake for 5 minutes in the preheated oven, then turn over and bake for another 5 to 10 minutes, until browned and crispy.

BURGERS FROM THE RANCH

Tablespoons: Eight - 15 minutes for preparation, 10 minutes for cooking, a total of 25 minutes. FACTS ABOUT DIET AND FITNESS

268, Carbohydrate 7, Fat 15, Protein 23, Protein 23, Cholesterol 98 mg. Calories 268, Fat 7.7 G.

To make this dish, you'll need two pounds of lean ground beef, three quarters cup of crushed saltine crackers, one one-ounce packet of ranch dressing mix and one small onion.

DIRECTIONS

Grill at a high temperature before using.

Gather your ingredients in a bowl and begin to combine them. in the shape of

Patties of hamburger meat

Grill grates should be brushed with a little coating of oil. Grill patties for 5 minutes on each side or until done.

CREAM CHICKEN WITH DIJON TARRAGON

Servings: four. - Preparation: 15m - Cooking: 30m - Total: 45m - NUTRITIONAL DETAILS: 310.1 kcal, 2.1 g carbs, 27.7 g protein, and 120.3 mg cholesterol.

In order to make this dish, you will need the following ingredients: f 1 tablespoon butter f 1/2 cup heavy cream f 1 tablespoon olive oil f 1 tablespoon Dijon mustard f 4 skinless, boneless chicken breast halves f 2 tablespoons chopped tarragon DIRECTIONS

Using a medium-high heat, melt the butter and oil together in a large skillet. Place the chicken in the pan and season it with salt and pepper. Both sides are brown. Cook for another 15 minutes, covered, on medium heat, or until the chicken juices run clear. Keep warm in a separate location.

Scrape the brown pieces off the bottom of the pan with a spatula as you add the cream. Incorporate mustard and tarragon into the mixture. 5 minutes of stirring will bring the sauce to a thickening point. Replenish sauce in pan with chicken and toss to coat. Serve the chicken with the rest of the sauce drizzled over it.

Burgers with spicy chipotle turkey are on the menu this week.

Servings: four. - 25 minutes for preparation, 10 minutes for cooking, a total of 35 minutes. 376 calories, 25.8 grams of carbohydrates, 15.3 grams of fat, 33.3 grams of protein, and 102 milligrams of cholesterol.

3 cups finely chopped onion 1 teaspoon onion powder 2 tablespoons chopped fresh cilantro 1/4 teaspoon black pepper 2 tablespoons chopped fresh cilantro 4 slices

mozzarella cheese 1 teaspoon garlic powder 4 hamburger buns, split and toast

DIRECTIONS

Lightly oil the grates of an outdoor grill and prepare it for medium-high heat. In a large bowl, combine the ground turkey, onion, and seasonings.

Chipotle chile peppers and cilantro are combined in a mixing bowl; add garlic powder, onion powder, seasoned salt and black pepper to taste. Make four patties out of the mixture.

Grill the hamburgers until the turkey is no longer pink in the middle, approximately 4 minutes each side. 2 minutes before they are done cooking, top the patties with the mozzarella pieces. Toast the buns before serving.

CHILI CON CHICKEN AND CORN

How many portions are there? Cooking time: 12 hours and 15 minutes. CALORIES: 187.9, Carbohydrates: 22.6g, Protein: 20.4g, Cholesterol: 40.6mg. A 16-ounce container of salsa, 1/4 teaspoon powdered black pepper, 2 teaspoons garlic powder, and 4 skinless, boneless chicken breast halves are all that's needed for this recipe.

Mexican-style corn, pinto beans, ground cumin, and chili powder f 1 (11-ounce) can of Mexican-style corn DIRECTIONS

The night before you intend to enjoy this chili, put the chicken and salsa in the slow cooker. Garlic is a great addition to any dish.

salt, pepper, cumin, and chili powder powder. On the Low setting, cook for 6 to 8 hours.

Shred the chicken with two forks about three to four hours before you plan to eat. Continue cooking the meat by putting it back in the pot.

Corn and pinto beans go into the slow cooker at this point. Cook until you're ready to serve, then remove from heat and serve immediately.

VEGETARIAN BURGERS MADE FROM HOME-MADE BLACK BEANS

Servings: four. - Preparation: 15m - Cooking: 20m - Total: 35m - FACTS ABOUT DIET AND FITNESS

Caloric intake: 198 kcal; macronutrient composition: 33.1g carbohydrate, 3g fat, 11.2g protein; cholesterol concentration: 46.1mg

1 (16-ounce) can washed and drained black beans 1 tablespoon chili powder 1/2 green bell pepper sliced into 2-inch chunks 1 tablespoon cumin 1/2 onion wedged 1 teaspoon Thai chili sauce or spicy sauce 3 peeled garlic cloves 1/2 cup bread crumbs 1 egg INTERNATIONAL INGREDIENTS

DIRECTIONS

Pre-heat an outside grill to high heat and lightly oil a piece of aluminum foil if you're going to be grilling it. When it comes to baking,

A baking sheet can be lightly oil and the oven preheated to 375°F (190°C).

Mash the black beans with a fork in a medium bowl until they are thick and pasty.

Finely chop the bell pepper, onion, and garlic in a food processor. Add to mashed beans and mix well.

Combine the egg, chili powder, cumin, and chili sauce in a small bowl.

Mix the crushed beans with the egg mixture. Make sure the mixture is sticky and holds together by adding bread crumbs at this point. Make four patties out of the mixture.

It takes roughly 8 minutes each side to cook burgers when using aluminum foil. You may cook patties either by placing them on a baking sheet or by broiling them for approximately 10 minutes on each side.

COOKED PORK SUBSTITUTES

The number of servings is 12 Preparation: 15 minutes - Cooking: 4h30 minutes - Total: 4h45 minutes NUTRITIONAL

DETAILS: 355 calories, 15.2 grams of carbohydrate, 18.1 grams of fat, and 30.2 grams of protein.

3 pounds of boneless pork ribs f 1 (14 ounce) can of beef broth f 1 (18 ounce) bottle of barbecue sauce

DIRECTIONS

Add boneless pork ribs and a can of beef stock to the slow cooker. 4 hours on high heat, or

For as long as the meat shreds with ease. Shred the meat with two forks after removing it. It may not seem to work immediately away, but it will.

Make sure the oven is preheated to 350 degrees Fahrenheit (175 degrees C). Shred the pork and add it to a dutch oven or iron skillet with barbeque sauce and mix well.

30 minutes in a preheated oven or until well cooked.

Garlic and lime chicken with a spicy kick.

Servings: four. - Preparation: 5m - Cooking: 20m - Total: 25m - 220 calories, 2.4 grams of carbohydrates, 10.7 grams of fat, 27.7 grams of protein, 8.4 mg of cholesterol and 84 milligrams of sodium

1/4teaspoon black pepper 1/4teaspoon dried parsley f 4 boneless, skinless chicken breast halves Add 1/8 teaspoon paprika to 1 tablespoon olive oil and 1/4 teaspoon garlic powder to 2 teaspoons garlic powder to 3 tablespoons lime juice and 1/4 teaspoon dried thyme to make this spicy and flavorful sauce. Use the ingredients listed in order.

DIRECTIONS Combine salt, black pepper, cayenne, paprika, and 1/4 teaspoon of garlic powder in a small bowl. Add onion and stir until well combined.

dried thyme, parsley, and pepper. Chicken breasts should be liberally coated in the spice mixture.

Over medium heat, melt the butter and olive oil in a large heavy skillet. Cook the chicken for 6 minutes on each side or until it is golden brown. Pour in 2 tablespoons of lime juice and 2 teaspoons of garlic powder. Cook for another 5 minutes, stirring often, to ensure that the sauce is uniformly coated.

MAC AND CHEESE IS CHUCK'S FAVORITE.

How many portions are there? - Preparation: 10 minutes - Cooking: 45 minutes - Total: 55 minutes - Count 591 calories, 45.5g carbohydrates, 33.3g fat, 26.8g protein, 88mg cholesterol

THE INGREDIENTS f1 (8 ounce) 1/4 cup of shredded Parmesan cheese f 1 box of elbow macaroni (8 ounce) sharply shredded package To taste, add salt and pepper to the cheddar cheese (12 ounce) little curd cottage cheese container f 1 cup dry crumbs of bread (8 ounce) 1/4 cup melted butter in a sour cream container DIRECTIONS

Make sure the oven is preheated to 350 degrees Fahrenheit (175 degrees C). As soon as a big pot of lightly salted water comes to a rolling boil, add the

Cook the pasta until al dente; drain well.

Macaroni and cheese, cottage cheese, sour cream, Parmesan cheese, and salt and pepper are mixed together in a 9x13-inch baking dish. Bake at 350 degrees Fahrenheit for 30 minutes. A little bowl of breadcrumbs and warmed butter is all that is needed to make this dish delicious. Over the macaroni mixture, sprinkle the topping.

Top should be golden brown after 30 to 35 minutes of baking.

BUTTER CHICKEN, A WORLD-FAMED FOOD

Servings: four. - 15 minutes for prep; 40 minutes for cooking; a total of 55 minutes. FACTS ABOUT DIET AND FITNESS

Calories: 447.5, Carbohydrates: 9.3g, Protein: 31.6g, Cholesterol: 222.6mg...

Chopped buttery round cracker crumbs, 4 skinless and boneless chicken breast halves, a bit of coarse black pepper, and 1/2 cup of butter are all that's needed to make this dish.

DIRECTIONS

Set the oven temperature to 375 degrees Fahrenheit (190 Celsius) (190 degrees C).

Two shallow dishes, one for the eggs and the other for the cracker crumbs, should be used. Garlic salt and cracker crumbs are combined in a bowl.

pepper. After dipping the chicken in the eggs, coat it with the crumb mixture.

Bake the coated chicken in a 9x13-inch baking dish at 350 degrees Fahrenheit for 30 minutes. Put butter on the chicken and serve.

Bake for 40 minutes, or until the chicken is no longer pink and the juices run clear, in a preheated oven.

Chicken Noodle Soup That's Quick and Easy

How many portions are there? Total preparation time is 30 minutes. FACTS ABOUT DIET AND FITNESS

Carbohydrates: 12.1g ; Protein: 13.4g ; Cholesterol: 46.4mg ; Total: 161.5 calories.

1/2 pound chopped cooked chicken breasts f 1 tablespoon butter 1 1/2 cups egg noodles f 1 cup chopped onion 1 cup cut carrots 1/2 teaspoon dried basil 1 cup chopped celery 2 cans of chicken broth 2 cans vegetable broth salt and pepper to taste

DIRECTIONS 1. Melt butter in a large saucepan over medium heat. The onion and celery should be just soft, about 5 minutes in the butter.

minutes. Chicken, noodles, carrots, basil oregano, salt and pepper are added to the chicken and vegetable broths. Then decrease the heat and simmer for around 20 minutes.

Baked Garlic Parmesan Chicken Recipe

How many portions are there? - Preparation: 15m - Cooking: 30m - Total: 45m - It has 281.1 calories, 13.7 grams of carbohydrates, 30.4 grams of protein, and 75 milligrams of cholesterol.

FILLING: 2 tablespoons of olive oil, 1 teaspoon of dried basil, 1 minced garlic clove, 1/4 teaspoon of powdered black pepper, 1 cup of dry bread crumbs, 6 skinless, boneless chicken breast halves, and 3/4 cup of grated Parmesan cheese; SERVING: 4 DIRECTIONS

Start by preheating the oven to 350°F (175 degrees C). A 9x13-inch baking dish should be lightly sprayed with cooking spray before use. 2. Combine the oil and garlic in a bowl. Mix the bread crumbs, Parmesan cheese, and garlic powder in a separate basin.

the two main ingredients are basil and black pepper. Using a bread crumbs and oil combination, coat each chicken breast in the breadcrumbs. Stack the bread crumbs on top of the chicken breasts in the baking dish and bake. To ensure that the chicken is cooked through and the fluids flow clear, bake for 30 minutes at the specified temperature.

GEORGE'S CHILI IS A CLASSIC.

At least ten. - 10 minutes for prep; 1 hour and 45 minutes for cooking; 1 hour and 55 minutes total. FACTS ABOUT DIET AND FITNESS

305 calories, 25.5 grams of carbohydrates, 13.7 grams of fat, 22.3 grams of protein, and 55 milligrams of cholesterol.

ingredients: 2 pounds lean ground beef, 1/8 teaspoon cayenne pepper, 1 can (46 fluid ounces), 1/2 teaspoon white sugar, 1 (29 ounce) 2 tablespoons of canned tomato sauce (15 ounce) 2 tablespoons of ground black pepper f 1 tablespoon of canned kidney beans (15 ounce) 1 1/2 cups chopped onion f 1 1/2 teaspoons ground cumin f 1/4 cup chopped green bell pepper f 1/4 cup chili powder f can pinto beans, drained and rinsed DIRECTIONS

Grease a large pan and add the meat. Cook until golden brown all over over a medium-high flame.

Dispose of and drain

crumble.

On high heat in a big pot mix the ground beef with tomato juice and tomato sauce as well as kidney beans and pinto beans as well as onions, bell peppers as well as cayenne pepper as well as sugar and oregano. Increase heat to high, then lower to medium-low. 1 and a half hours of simmering is plenty. Cook on low for 8 to 10 hours in a slow cooker, according to the manufacturer's instructions.)

RICE FROM MEXICO

Servings per recipe: four Preparation: 5 minutes - Cooking: 25 minutes - Total: 30 minutes - Count Facts about nutrition

Nutritional information for this meal includes 291, Carbohydrates (42.4), Fat (11), Protein (4.8), and cholesterol (3/3) mg.

INGREDIENTS\sf Fry 3 tbsp of veg oil Frozen onion cubes long-grain rice, 1 cup raw, uncooked Tomato sauce in a half cup Fifteen milligrams of garlic powder 2 mugs of chicken stock f 1/8 teaspoon cumin seed powder

DIRECTIONS

Set up an oil and rice pan in a big pot over medium heat. When the mixture has puffed up, remove it from the heat.

golden. Salt and cumin may be added to the rice while it's cooking.

Toss in the onions and sauté for a few minutes until they are soft. Bring to a boil, then add the tomato sauce and chicken broth.

Simmer for 20 to 25 minutes with the heat down to low and the lid on. Fluff with a fork

APPLESAUCE FROM SARAH

Servings per recipe: four Total time spent in the kitchen: 30 minutes. Nutrition Facts: 121 calories, 31.8 grams of carbohydrates, 0.2 grams of fat, 0.4 grams of protein, and 0mg of cholesterol.

1/4 cup white sugar, 1/2 teaspoon ground cinnamon, 4 cored and diced apples, 3/4 cup water

DIRECTIONS

1. In a saucepan, add apples, water, sugar, and cinnamon.
2. Bring to a boil, then reduce the heat and simmer for 30 minutes. Over medium heat, cover with a lid and cook for 15 to 20 minutes

The apples should be tender in around 20 minutes. Mash with a potato masher or fork when it's cooled down.

Chicken Baked with Honey Mustard

Servings: six Total time spent in the kitchen: 1 hour and 15 minutes. It has 232 calories, 24.8g of carbohydrates, 25.6g protein, 67.1mg of Cholesterol per serving.

INGREDIENTS: 6 skinless, boneless chicken breast halves 1 teaspoon dried basil 1 teaspoon paprika 1 teaspoon honey 1/2 cup dry parsley 1/2 cup prepared mustard 1 teaspoon DIRECTIONS

Make sure the oven is preheated to 350 degrees Fahrenheit (175 degrees C).

In a 9x13-inch baking dish, season the chicken breasts with salt and pepper to taste.

dish. Mix the honey, mustard, basil, paprika, and parsley in a small bowl. Make sure everything is well-combined. Brush the chicken with the remaining half of the sauce once it has been poured over it.

Bake for 30 minutes at 375 degrees Fahrenheit in an oven that has been preheated. Brush the other side of the chicken with the rest of the honey mustard mix. The chicken should no longer be pink and the juices should flow clear after a further 10 to 15 minutes in the oven. Allow 10 minutes of cooling time before serving.

Chick-fil-A CHICKEN

Servings per recipe: four - Preparation: 10 minutes - Cooking: 30 minutes - Total: 40 minutes - Count Facts about nutrition

calories: 548.5; carbohydrates: 13.1g; protein: 34.4"

INGREDIENTS

3 cups grated Parmesan cheese f 4 skinless, boneless chicken breasts f 3/4 cup mayonnaise 1 can artichoke hearts, drained and chopped 1 pinch of garlic pepper

DIRECTIONS

The oven should be preheated at 375 degrees Fahrenheit (190 degrees C).

Mix the artichoke hearts, Parmesan cheese, mayonnaise, and garlic powder in a medium-sized mixing basin.

Cover the chicken evenly with the artichoke mixture in a greased baking dish.

In a preheated oven, cook the chicken for 30 minutes, or until it's no longer pink in the middle and the juices flow clear.

CASSEROLE WITH CHICKEN FLORENTINE

Servings per recipe: four Preparation: 25m - Cooking: 25m - Total: 50m. There are 646.7 calories, 17.6 grams of carbohydrate, and 61.6 grams of protein in this meal.

The following ingredients can be used to make this dish: 4 skinless, boneless chicken breasts, 1/2 cup half-and-half, 1/4 cup butter, 1/2 cup Parmesan cheese, 3 teaspoons minced garlic, 2 (13.5-ounce) cans of drained spinach, 1 tablespoon lemon juice, 4 ounces of sliced fresh mushrooms, 1 (10.75-ounce) can condensed cream of mushroom soup, 2/3 cup bacon bits, 1 tablespoon Italian seasoning, and 2 cups shredded mozzarella cheese

The oven should be preheated at 350 degrees Fahrenheit (175 degrees C). The chicken breast halves should be baked on a baking pan.

In the range of 20-30 minutes, until the liquid is no longer pink and the pulp is completely removed. Remove from the heat and let to cool. Add a 400-degree Fahrenheit temperature increase to the oven temperature (200 degrees C).

In a medium saucepan, melt the butter over medium heat. Toss the garlic and lemon into the mixture and keep going.

Italian spice, half-and-half, and grated Parmesan cheese round out the recipe. 4. Cover the bottom of a 9x9-inch baking dish with spinach. Mushrooms may be used to cover up the spinach.

The mushrooms should be covered with half of the remaining mixture. Place the chicken breasts in the dish and pour the remaining sauce mixture over them. Mozzarella cheese and bacon pieces are the finishing touches. 5. Bake at 400 degrees F (200 degrees C) for 20 to 25 minutes, until bubbling and golden.

PASTA CASSEROLE DEL MONTE

Servings Per Recipe: 6 Cooks: 20 minutes; 15 minutes for preparation; 35 minutes for the whole process. Nutrition information

595 calories, 58.1 grams of carbohydrates, 26.1 grams of fat, 32.1 grams of protein, and 99 milligrams of cholesterol.

FEATURES f 1 (12 ounce) package egg noodles f 2 cans of tuna drained f 1/4 cup chopped onion 10.5 ounces of condensed cream of mushroom soup 2 cups of shredded Cheddar cheese 1 cup of frozen green peas 1 cup of crushed potato chips

DIRECTIONS

Bring a big saucepan of water to a boil with a little salt. Drain the pasta and return it to the pot of boiling water.

The oven should be preheated at 425 degrees Fahrenheit (220 degrees C).

Cook pasta according to package directions; drain and rinse under cold water until al dente; drain well. In a 9x13-inch baking dish, combine the remaining 1 cup of cheese with the potato chip crumbs.

Once the oven has been warmed, bake for 15 to 20 minutes, or until the cheese has melted.

CHICKEN BLEU

Food for four people - Preparation: 10m - Cooking: 35m - Total: 45m - Nutrition information

There are 418.8 calories, 12.6 grams of carbohydrates, 46.1 grams of protein, and 123.6 milligrams of cholesterol in a serving of this dish.

SUGGESTED INGREDIENTS: 4 skinless, boneless chicken breast halves; 6 slices of Swiss cheese; 1/4 teaspoon salt; 4 slices of cooked ham; 1/8 teaspoon black pepper; 1/2 cup of bread crumbs; seasonings; DIRECTIONS

The oven should be preheated at 350 degrees Fahrenheit (175 degrees C). Prepare a 7-by-11-inch baking dish by spraying it with nonstick spray.

spray.

Pound the chicken breasts to 1/4-inch thickness.

Salt and pepper each piece of chicken on both sides before cooking it. Place a piece of cheese and a slice of ham on top of each chicken breast. You may fasten each breast by wrapping it around a toothpick. Place the chicken in a baking dish and equally coat it with bread crumbs.

30 to 35 minutes in the oven, or until no longer pink. Remove from the oven and top each breast with half a cheddar slice. The cheese should be melted, so put it back in for another 3 to 5 minutes. Serve immediately once toothpicks have been removed.

Chips made with baked kale

Servings Per Recipe: 6 - Preparation: 10m - Cooking: 10m - Total: 20m Nutrition information

Fat: 2.8g, Protein: 2.5g, and Cholesterol: 0mg per serving.

INGREDIENTS: 1 bunch kale, 1 tbsp. olive oil, and 1 tsp. seasoned salt.

A 350-degree Fahrenheit oven is the ideal temperature for this recipe (175 degrees C). parchment paper on a cookie sheet that is not insulated

paper.

Make bite-sized pieces by tearing the leaves off the thick stems with a knife or kitchen scissors. Using a salad spinner, completely dry the kale. Toss the kale with a little olive oil and salt to taste.

Ten to fifteen minutes should be enough time to brown the edges but not burn them.

BETTER TUNA MELT (NEW JERSEY DINER STYLE)

Food for four people Prepare: 10m Cooks: 5m - Total time: 15m Nutrition information

484 calories, 22.1g carbohydrates, 28.4g fat, 34.8g protein, and 76mg cholesterol in a serving of chicken

INGREDIENTS

4 slices seedless rye bread f 1 1/2 teaspoons finely chopped onion f 8 slices of ripe tomato f 1 tablespoon chopped parsley f 3/4 teaspoon of red wine vinegar f paprika, for garnish DIRECTIONS

Turn on the broiler on your oven.

A bowl should be used to combine the tuna with mayonnaise and other ingredients such as celery and onion as well as the vinegar. Salt and pepper your food to taste. 3) Broil the rye bread slices on a baking sheet in the oven for one minute to toast the bread.

toasted. Remove from the heat and top with the tuna salad before removing from the oven. Layer tuna salad with 1 cheese slice, 1 tomato slice, and the remaining cheese pieces on top of each piece of toast. If you'd like, you may broil it for a few minutes to melt the cheese on the bread.

Vegetable Stir-Fry with Ginger

Servings Per Recipe: 6 Preparation: 25 minutes - Cooking: 15 minutes - Total: 40 minutes Nutrient Facts: 119 calories, 8 grams of carbs, 9.3 grams of fat, 2.2 grams of protein, and 0mg of cholesterol in a serving.

INGREDIENTS f 1 tablespoon cornstarch f 3/4 cup julienned carrots f f 2 tablespoons of minced fennel F 2 tablespoons soy sauce and 1/4 cup vegetable oil, split f 2 teaspoons chopped fresh ginger root 1 small head of broccoli, chopped into florets f 2 1/2 teaspoons of water Half a cup snow peas f 1 tablespoon salt f 1/4 cup finely sliced onion Cornstarch, garlic, 1 teaspoon of ginger, and 2 tablespoons of vegetable oil should be blended in a large basin until they form a smooth paste.

The cornstarch has been dispersed. Slightly stir the vegetables with a fork before serving. Over medium-high heat, add the remaining 2 tablespoons of oil to a large pan or wok. Two minutes of steady stirring is all that is needed to avoid overcooking the veggies in the oil. Incorporate water and soy sauce. Make a paste by adding onion, salt, and 1 teaspoon of leftover ground ginger. Cook until the veggies are soft but not mushy, but not mushy.

SALAD DE FIESTA DE CHICKEN (CHILI)

Food for four people The total cooking time is 40 minutes: 10 minutes for prepping, 30 minutes for the actual cooking, and 10 minutes for cleanup. Nutrition information

310.8 calories, 42.2 grams of carbohydrate, 23.3 grams of protein, and 35.9 milligrams of cholesterol per serving.

1 (1.27 ounce) dry fajita seasoning packet divided into 2 equal portions 2 skinless, boneless chicken breasts 1 (10 ounce) package mixed salad greens 1 tablespoon vegetable oil 2 (15.5 ounce) cans rinsed and drained black beans 2 (11.1-ounce) canned Mexican-style corn 2 (10.5-ounce) cans cut into wedges 3 (3-ounce) cans diced jalapenos

DIRECTIONS

Toss half the fajita seasoning with the chicken and coat it evenly. Using a medium-high heat, sauté the onion in oil until translucent.

For 8 minutes on each side, or until the juices run clear, remove the chicken and set it aside.

Pour all of the ingredients into a large saucepan and bring to a boil over medium-high heat. Heat to a comfortable temperature by stirring occasionally over a medium flame.

Salad is ready when you toss the greens, onion, and tomato together. Dress salad with bean and corn dressing and top with chicken.

SEASONED CHICKEN BREASTS

Food for four people - 15 minutes for preparation; 15 minutes for cooking; a total of 30 minutes. Fat: 9.2g; carbs: 9.2g; protein: 29.5g; cholesterol: 68 mmol/dL

This recipe includes the following ingredients: 2 1/2 tablespoons paprika (flour, sugar, salt, and spices), 1 teaspoon dried thyme, 2 teaspoons garlic powder, one teaspoon ground cayenne pepper, one teaspoon salt, and one teaspoon ground black pepper.

DIRECTIONS

Garlic powder, onion powder, thyme and cayenne pepper are all mixed together in a medium bowl with the paprika.

plus freshly ground black pepper. You'll only need a small amount for the chicken, so keep it in an airtight container for future use (for seasoning fish, meats, or vegetables).

Prepare a medium-high-heat grill by preheating it. Rub some of the remaining 3 tablespoons of seasoning on both sides of the chicken breasts.

Grill grates should be brushed with a light coating of oil. The juices should run clear when the chicken is cooked for 6 to 8 minutes per side on the grill.

Tender, flavorful breasts of chicken basted in a flavorful herb sauce.

Food for four people Preparation: 15 minutes - Cooking: 45 minutes - Total: 1 hour Nutrition information

Meat: 45.1g; Protein: 1.1g; Cholesterol: 126.6mg; Calories: 391.5

The following ingredients should be added to your recipe: 3 tablespoons of extra virgin olive oil, 1/4 teaspoon of dried marjoram, 1 tablespoon of minced onion, 1/2 teaspoon salt, one clove of crushed garlic, 1/2 teaspoon of freshly ground black pepper, 1 teaspoon of dried thyme, 1/8 teaspoon of hot pepper sauce, and 1/2 teaspoon of crushed dried rosemary. Skinless bone-in chicken breast halves, 4 Chopped fresh parsley with a quarter teaspoon of finely ground sage

DIRECTIONS

The oven should be preheated at 425 degrees Fahrenheit (220 degrees C).

Salted and peppered chicken breasts will benefit from a basting sauce made with olive oil and an assortment of fresh herbs and spices.

The chicken breasts should be thoroughly coated with the sauce. Using a shallow baking dish, place the skin-side-up. Cover.

While basting frequently with pan drippings, roast for about 35 to 45 minutes at 425 degrees F (220 degrees C). Serve immediately on a warm platter, garnished with fresh parsley and any remaining pan juices.

BRUSCHETTA CHICKEN BAKE IN A JETT

Servings Per Recipe: 6 50m - Preparation: 20m - Cooks: 30m - Nutrition information

There are 230 calories in this meal; 8.2 grams of carbohydrates; 9.4 grams of fat; 21 grams of protein; 41 milligrams of cholesterol;

This recipe calls for 1 1/2 pounds of cubed skinless, boneless chicken breast halves, along with 1 tablespoon minced garlic, 1 teaspoon salt, and a 6-ounce box of chicken-flavored dry bread stuffing mix. Also included are 2 cups shredded mozzarella cheese, half a cup of water, and 1 tablespoon Italian seasoning, as well as 1 tablespoon of garlic powder.

DIRECTIONS

First, heat the oven to 400 degrees F. (200 degrees C). Cooking spray a 9x13-inch glass baking dish is all you need for this recipe. A large bowl of cubed chicken and salt should be used for this purpose. The chicken should be arranged in a single layer at the bottom of the pan.

An oven-safe dish. In a large bowl, combine the tomatoes, water, garlic, and stuffing mix; set aside to soften for about 30 minutes. Sprinkle the cheese on top of the chicken, and then add the Italian seasoning to the mixture. Spread the softened stuffing mixture over the top.

3. Bake until the chicken is no longer pink in the center, about 30 minutes, with the lid off.